Key Topics in Brain Research

Edited by
A. Carlsson, P. Riederer, H. Beckmann, T. Nagatsu,
S. Gershon, and K. A. Jellinger

SpringerWienNewYork

G. Wieselmann (ed.)

Current Update in Psychoimmunology

SpringerWienNewYork

Prof. Dr. G. Wieselmann
Psychiatrische Universitätsklinik,
LKH Graz, Graz, Austria

© 1997 Springer-Verlag/Wien
Reprint of the original edition 1997

Product Liability: The publisher can give no guarantee for information about drug dosage and application thereof contained in this book. In every individual case the respective user must check its accuracy by consulting other pharmaceutical literature. The use of registered names, trademarks, etc. in this publication does not imply, even in the absence of a specific statement, that such names are exempt from the relevant protective laws and regulations and therefore free for general use.

Typesetting: H.-D. Ecker Textverarbeitung, D-53225 Bonn

Graphic design: Ecke Bonk
Printed on acid-free and chlorine-free bleached paper
SPIN: 10634039

With 16 Figures

ISSN 0934–1420
ISBN-13: 978-3-211-83029-1   e-ISBN-13: 978-3-7091-6870-7
DOI: 10.1007/978-3-7091-6870-7

Preface

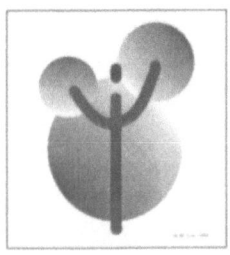

This book is based on lectures held at the International Expert Meeting "Current Update on Psychoimmunology" (September 26–28, 1996, Graz, Austria), which was organized by "Verein zur Förderung der Wissenschaft und Forschung an der Universitätsklinik für Psychiatrie Graz" (Chairman: H.-G. Zapotoczky; Coordinators: M. Lux, G. Wieselmann; Local Organizing Committee: E. Braun, M. Bretterklieber, H. Häusler, G. Herzog, S. Kriechbaum, S. Sperlich). The book tries to close the gap between immunological findings on one hand, psychological, psychopathological, electrophysiological and neuroimaging aspects on the other. It also deals with the issue of "cause and effect" (of immunological alternatives) in different organic and/or mental disorders, and emphasizes the necessity of considering a variety of treatment strategies. There are dynamic interactions and several important similarities between the immune system and the central nervous system, which help to lay the rational basis for "psychoimmunology". Both systems have the capacity for memory and both play vital roles in adaptation and defence. Furthermore, in each system pathological changes can occur in the event of inappropriate responses to internal or external stimuli, leading to psychiatric as well as organic illnesses and autoimmune diseases could also arise as a consequence of dysfunction and maladaptation, respectively.

Finally, the editor is grateful to all the authors and experts for their contributions to the meeting and for preparing their manuscripts for this publication.

Graz, November 1997   G. WIESELMANN

Contents

Psychoimmunology: basic research and an integrative view

Kaschka, W. P.: Psychoneuroimmunology and neuroendocrinology – an integrative view 1

Schauenstein, K., Rinner, I., Felsner, P., Liebmann, P., Haas, H. S., Hofer, D., Wölfler, A., Korsatko, W.: The role of the autonomous nervous system in the dialogue between the brain and immune system 13

Sun, Y., Yolken, R., Stanley Neuropathology Consortium: Analysis of gene expression of human brain 23

Tilz, G. P., Demel, U., Wieselmann, G., Fabisch, H., Zapotoczky, H. G., Wachter, H., Fuchs, D.: New trends in neuropsychiatry: polyimmunotherapy – a new way of treatment in neurology and psychiatry. The 5S–7S Tilz protocol and the antigen clearing deficiency syndromes 29

Schizophrenia: immunological measurements

Fabisch, H., Fabisch, K., Zapotoczky, H. G., Tilz, G. P., Langs, G., Demel, U., Wieselmann, G.: Immunological alterations in three types of schizophrenia 35

Ganguli, R.: Cytokine abnormalities in schizophrenia: a review of their pathogenic significance, with particular reference to the autoimmune hypothesis 39

van Kammen, D. P., McAllister, C. G., Kelley, M. E.: Relationship between immune and behavioral measures in schizophrenia 51

Müller, N., Riedel, M., Schwarz, M., Gruber, R., Ackenheil, M.: Immunomodulatory effects of neuroleptics to the cytokine system and the cellular immune system in schizophrenia 57

Rothermundt, M., Arolt, V., Weitzsch, C., Eckhoff, D., Kirchner, H.: Cytokines in schizophrenia. Results from a longitudinal study 69

Immunological aspects in mental disorders and Alzheimer's disease

Langs, G., Herzog, G., Penkner, K., Demel, U., Tilz, G., Bratschko, R. O., Wieselmann, G.: Psychoimmunology, anxiety disorders and TMJ-disorders 79

Lemke, M. R., Glatzel, M., Henneberg, A. E.: Immunological alterations and neuropsychiatric symptoms: antimicroglia antibodies and psychopathological subgroups in Alzheimer's disease 85

Schott, K., Schnaidt, M., Batra, A., Bartels, M., Buchkremer, G.: Platelet antibodies in mental disorder   93

Schott, K., Batra, A., Uhl, A., Bartels, M., Buchkremer, G.: Plasma levels of interleukin 1β and interleukin 6 in mental disorders   99

Electrobiophysiological and neuroimaging aspects

Born, J., Späth-Schwalbe, E.: Effects of cytokines on human EEG and sleep   103

Catafau, A. M., Parellada, E., Lomeña, F., Bernardo, M.: Role of cingulate gyrus during Wisconsin card sorting test: a single photon emission computed tomography (SPECT) study   119

Psychoneuroimmunology and neuroendocrinology – an integrative view

W. P. Kaschka

Abteilung Psychiatrie I, Universität Ulm, und Zentrum für Psychiatrie
Weissenau, Ravensburg-Weissenau, Federal Republic of Germany

Some historical aspects on the development of psychoneuroimmunology

A paper with the title "Infectio psychica" was published as early as 1846 in the Österreichische Medizinische Wochenschrift (Austrian Weekly Medical Journal) (Hofbauer, 1846). Hofbauer speculated that psychiatric illnesses may possibly be transmitted by infection. This hypothesis was also adopted by others in the following decades, e.g. by Baillarger (1857) and Wollenberg (1889). This approach was further pursued by various authors in the 20th century: a virus hypothesis was formulated to explain endogenous psychoses (for review see Kaschka, 1989). Three major strategies of research resulted from this hypothesis:

1. Antibody studies in serum and CSF with a view to detecting local (autochthonous) immunoglobulin synthesis in the central nervous system (CNS).
2. Detection of intact viruses, viral nucleic acid or viral antigens in brain tissue (biopsy or autopsy material) or CSF.
3. Investigations on transmission to experimental animals using brain tissue or CSF.

The results obtained with these strategies were compiled by Kaschka (1989). Developments in recent years are also described by Taller et al. (1996) and by Henneberg and Kaschka (1997).

Influences of the CNS on immune processes were investigated scientifically for the first time by Bogendörfer (1927). Further developments in this area of research will be described in more detail below.

Bidirectional interactions between the central nervous system and the immune system

All immunologically important organs in humans such as the thymus, spleen, lymph nodes and bone marrow are innervated by the autonomic nervous system.

At present, little is known about the functional significance of this innervation. However, recent experimental findings support the view that the autonomic nervous system has regulatory effects on lymphatic organs (reviews at Kaschka and Aschauer, 1990; Ader et al., 1991; Husband, 1993). It could be shown that inhibitory effects on immune reactions are mediated by sympathetic nerve fibers. If for example the spleen is denervated in animal experiments, immune reactions are stimulated. This is evidently based on the removal of inhibitory influences. Conversely, immunosuppression can be demonstrated after administration of alpha-adrenergic agonists. These are by no means one-way processes, but bidirectional interactions as shown by the fall in the noradrenaline content of the spleen after immunization of experimental animals with a standard antigen, e.g. sheep erythrocytes (Besedovsky et al., 1985).

Further evidence for the close interrelationship between the nervous system and the immune system has been provided by modern immunohistochemical techniques. It was thus possible to identify neurotransmitters and their specific binding sites (receptors) in numerous lymphoid tissues. For example, noradrenergic receptors (mainly beta receptors) are found in lymph nodes. This may be considered as further evidence documenting a regulatory function of the noradrenergic system in lymphocyte activity and possibly also in lymphocyte maturation. Some authors assume that the humoral immune response (antibody production) can be stimulated as a result of inhibition of the activity of T suppressor cells by beta adrenergic impulses. There are various experimental findings to support the assumption that besides the beta-adrenergic system, the alpha-adrenergic, the serotoninergic and the dopaminergic systems may also have immunomodulatory capacity.

Knowledge of the neuroanatomical basis of the interactions between the nervous system and the immune system is still quite incomplete. However, thanks to the availability of highly differentiated methods of investigation, it is becoming ever more extensive. The description of hitherto unknown neuronal links, e.g. that recently reported to connect the brainstem and the thymus is a visible result of these research endeavors (cf. Bulloch, 1985; Ader et al., 1991).

The discovery that regulatory impulses act on the immune system not only from the CNS (efferent arm), but that conversely information also passes from the immune system to the CNS (afferent arm) is of great importance. This means that there is a closed control loop in the cybernetic sense. Whereas many components of the efferent arm have already been known for a long time, the afferent arm was only in part characterized in recent years (Besedovsky et al., 1986). The hormones of the hypothalamopituitary-adrenal (HPA) axis mainly have immuno-suppressant effects in the periphery. Receptors for corticosteroids (but also for insulin, growth hormone, estradiol and testosterone) could be demonstrated on lymphoid cells.

Besides the glucocorticoids, androgens, estrogens and progesterone suppress the immune response in vivo, whereas growth hormone, thyroxine and insulin have an immunostimulant action. Prolactin also appears to play a role in immunomodulation. Receptors for this hormone could be detected on lymphocytes. Observations in patients with heart transplants indicate that the level of prolactin in the plasma is raised prior to a rejection reaction (Carrier et al., 1987).

The discovery and characterization of the afferent arm of the system began with the observation that substantially raised levels of glucocorticoids occurred in the plasma after immunization of experimental animals with standard antigens, e.g. sheep erythrocytes. Chronologically, the rises coincided in time with the peak immune response. This posed the question as to the existence of immunological signals which are recognized by neuroendocrine structures and which participate in the regulation of the plasma glucocorticoid level. This question could be investigated experimentally.

Besedovsky et al. (1981) were able to prove that stimulated lymphoid cells are the source of one or several factors which stimulate glucocorticoid secretion. The authors initially designated this newly discovered activity as "glucocorticoid increasing factor" (GIF). After hypophysectomy or administration of dexamethasone, an increase of corticosterone could no longer be attained by administration of GIF. However, the plasma glucocorticoids rise in intact untreated animals after intracerebroventricular injection of GIF. GIF probably acts in the hypothalamus. According to present knowledge, its effect is mediated by an increased release of corticotropin releasing factor (CRF).

Later investigations showed that GIF comprises substances from the cytokine group (cf. Brown and Blalock, 1991). The cytokines, which inter alia also include interleukin 1 (IL-1) which is involved in the development of fever, participate in the transmission of information between various lymphocytic and monocytic cell types. They evidently also fulfill the function of neurotransmitters or neuromodulators. In the example of the bidirectional interactions between the CNS and the immune system described above, "feedback" control of the immune response is ensured with the mediation of interleukins (GIF). This might be necessary to regulate the extent and duration of immune reactions once they have been triggered (Fig. 1).

The complexity of such regulatory processes is exceedingly great. It is therefore not surprising that other groups of neuromodulators also have effects on the immune system. For example, American researchers observed an increase in the activity of natural human killer cells (NK

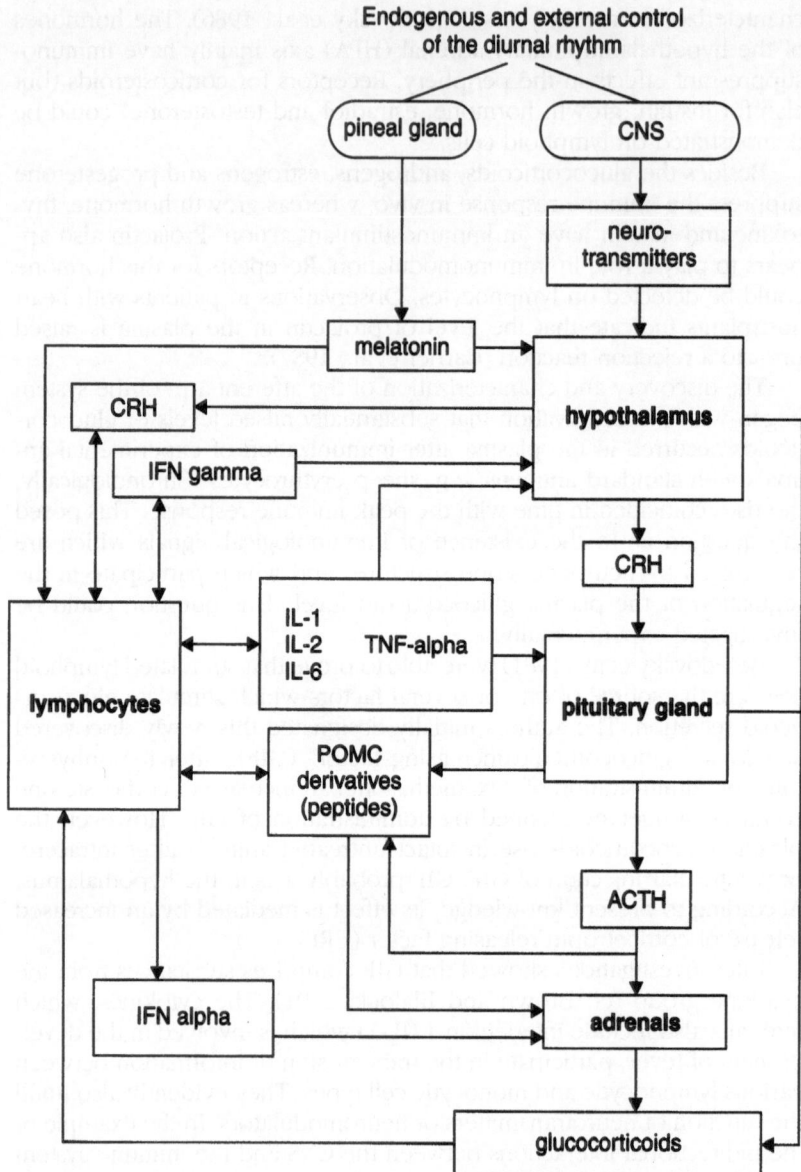

Fig. 1. Bidirectional interactions between the hypothalamopituitary-adrenal (HPA system) and the immune system (modified and supplemented according to Gatti et al., 1992), CRH: corticotropin releasing hormone, IL: interleukin, POMC: proopiomelanocortin, TNF: tumor necrosis factor, ACTH: adrenocorticotropic hormone, IFN: interferon

cells) in the presence of morphines and endogenous opioids, especially enkephalins. In most cases, these effects could be inhibited by the opiate antagonist naloxone (Wybran, 1985).

A further indication for the close functional link between the CNS and the immune system is the fact that after immunization alterations in the electrical activity of hypothalamic nuclei could be observed with sensitive electrophysiological techniques using intracerebral recordings in experimental animals. These changes in electrical activity were synchronous with the peak immune reaction (for review see Saphier and Ovadia, 1990).

Clinical relevance of psychoimmunological interactions

The practical relevance of the interaction between the CNS and the immune system was shown in the classic conditioning experiments of Ader and Cohen (1982). These authors demonstrated that immunosuppressant actions in the mouse can be conditioned under certain specific experimental conditions. First of all, they carried out immunosuppression by simultaneous administration of cyclophosphamide and saccharin. Under the selected experimental conditions, immunosuppressant effects could later be attained in the same mice by administration of saccharin alone (review at Kaschka and Aschauer, 1990, as well as Ader et al., 1991).

In recent years, there was great scientific interest in the influence of momentous life events (e.g. loss of the marriage partner) on various cellular immune functions in humans (McDaniel, 1992). A method of practical relevance for testing aspects of "immunocompetence" of the cellular immune system is the stimulation of cultured lymphocytes with lectins. Lectins are proteins of plant origin resembling antibodies. Some substances from this group have the property of preferentially activating T cells (e.g. phytohemagglutinin, PHA, and concanavalin A, Con A) or B cells (T cell-dependent, e.g. pokeweed mitogen, PWM). This activation is manifested as an increase of DNA synthesis which can be measured by the incorporation of ^{3}H-labeled thymidine (review at Stites, 1987). However, it should be noted that the clinical significance in particular of slight changes of activity is difficult to appraise in view of the complexity and susceptibility of this test system to interference. Clinical relevance can therefore not be directly inferred from data obtained with a single test method. This must also be taken into consideration in interpreting the investigations reported below.

In a study of Stein et al. (1985), 15 husbands of women with terminal breast cancer were investigated with regard to the stimulability of the blood lymphocytes with lectins before and after the death of their wives. A distinct fall in the stimulability of lymphocytes was shown immediately after the death of the wife. Follow-up examinations showed that this parameter rose again to the initial value after one year had elapsed.

Stein et al. (1985) also carried out investigations in depressive patients. Eighteen severely depressive inpatients were compared with a corresponding number of only slightly depressive outpatients, showing a significantly lower stimulability of lymphocytes of the peripheral blood in the first group relative to a healthy control group. However, the second group of patients did not show any difference from the control group.

A review of 12 studies on the stimulability of lymphocytes of the peripheral blood with the lectins phytohemagglutinin (PHA), concanavalin A (Con A), and pokeweed mitogen (PWM) in depressive patients revealed heterogenous findings (Stein and Trestman, 1990). Seven communications reported on a reduced stimulability of the lymphocytes with at least one lectin; in the remaining five studies, no change in stimulability was detected compared to the controls.

Differences in the characteristics of the patient populations and differences in methods are doubtless important factors which are able to explain the heterogeneity of the findings, at least in part.

Whereas Rapaport (1994) did not find any indication for activation of the immune system compared to a matched control group in patients with bipolar affective conditions who were in remission (i.e. who were euthymic), numerous results were found in patients with major depression during depressive phases. This indicated an activation of cell-mediated immunity (Maes, 1994). The findings included inter alia raised serum levels of the soluble interleukin 2 receptor (sIL-2R), positive acute phase proteins (Maes et al., 1995a) and a monocyte dysfunction (Cervera-Enguix and Rodriguez-Rosado, 1994). It was interesting that there were significant positive correlations of interleukin 6 (IL-6) and sIL-2R with cortisol in the plasma as well as between sIL-2R and prolactin in patients with major depression (Maes et al., 1995b).

In relatives of Alzheimer patients who were looking after the Alzheimer patients at home, Irwin et al. (1991) investigated the correlation of sympathetic tonus as a parameter of stress measured on the basis of the concentrations of adrenaline, noradrenaline and neuropeptide Y (NPY) in the serum on the one hand with the natural cytotoxicity (NK cell activity) on the other hand. They found a negative correlation between NPY concentration and the natural cytotoxicity, but no correlation between the NK cell activity and the concentrations of adrenaline and noradrenaline in the serum. This finding might be clinically relevant, since NK cells are involved in the recognition and destruction of virus-infected cells in the body.

In connection with diseases which are especially therapy-resistant, such as cancer conditions and AIDS, the significance of the way in which the individual copes with the disease has recently been the subject of a lively discussion. Some authors postulate a direct correlation between the patient's psychological coping with the disease and the prognosis. They attribute this to psychoimmunological mechanisms. However, we consider that great caution is called for, since the present findings are not capable of uniform interpretation (Cassileth et al., 1985; Rabkin et al., 1991; Perry et al., 1992; Goodkin et al., 1994). There is no question that the field of "psychooncology" referred to is an exceedingly interesting area of research from which important results may be expected.

It is clear from what has been stated above that the interactions between the central nervous system and the immune system involve an exceedingly complex meshwork of regulatory processes which we are only beginning to understand today. For a comprehensive understanding of the physiology and pathophysiology, it is particularly important to be aware that signals do not only pass from the CNS to the immune system, but that there is also an afferent arm which closes the control loop and via which information passes from the immune system into the CNS with mediation of cytokines. In this way, a complex network of regulatory processes arises which comprises the electrophysiological, the biochemical, the neuroendocrine and the immunological levels. This enables a bidirectional transmission of signals between structures of the central nervous system and components of the immune system.

Special immunological features in schizophrenic illnesses

Lines of argumentation supporting an autoimmune hypothesis to explain schizophrenia can be pursued at different levels: at the level of formal criteria of the disease course, there are numerous analogies between schizophrenia and classical autoimmunopathies, e.g. multiple sclerosis (MS) and systemic lupus erythematosus (SLE). All these illnesses can progress with flare-ups and remissions (often leaving behind residues), they can also have a chronic progressive course or be chronically progressive with additional flare-ups.

On the clinical level, there have been numerous reports that paranoid hallucinatory schizophreniform symptoms occur in classic autoimmune diseases (Kaschka, 1984; Lishman, 1987; Piesiur-Strehlow et al., 1988; Schiffer and Hoffman, 1991). However, it must be considered in the individual case whether this is most probably a (fortuitous?) coincidence of autoimmunopathy with an endogenous psychosis or alternatively an (endogenomorphic) psychosis of organic origin which is symptomatic of the involvement of the brain in the autoimmune disease. Factors in the history, especially chronological correlations between the occurrence of somatic and psychiatric symptoms, play an important role (cf. Kaschka, 1984).

On the other hand, it can be speculated that numerous postoperative psychoses of organic etiology occurring in particular after large-scale abdominal and thoracic operations with complications are mediated by

the release of cytokines. A similar situation is likely to obtain in respect
of organically induced psychoses in febrile patients. However, exact
elucidation of these processes must be left to future research work.

At the molecular or laboratory diagnostic level, numerous findings
were obtained at least in subgroups of schizophrenic patients. These
findings also occur with an increased incidence in classical autoimmunopathies and can consequently be regarded as (relatively) typical for this group of diseases. These include for example raised serum
concentrations of the soluble interleukin 2 receptor (sIL-2R, McAllister
et al., 1991; Rapaport and Lohr, 1994), changed rates of production of
IL-2 (Ganguli et al., 1992), raised numbers of autoantibody-producing
B cells (so-called CD5⁺ B lymphocytes, McAllister et al., 1991), an altered neopterin production (Sperner-Unterweger et al., 1992; neopterin
is a specific product of activated immune cells), the detection of autoantibodies in the serum (Galinowski et al., 1992; Chengappa et al., 1995)
and the detection of a shift in the ratio of the four immunoglobulin G
(IgG) subclasses in the serum (Kaschka et al., 1989).

Very largely, the relevance of these findings and their correlations
with clinical parameters have not yet been adequately elucidated today.
This will confront us with extensive research tasks in the future (cf.
Ganguli et al., 1992; Müller et al., 1993).

Besides the findings discussed up to now, which are generally interpreted as indicating the involvement of autoimmune processes, the
detection of antibodies and immune processes which are specifically
directed against brain structures and brain antigens are of particular
relevance. These are attributed a special role in the etiopathogenesis
of schizophrenia (e.g. receptors for dopamine or glutamate; review at
Kaschka, 1985a; cf. also Schott et al., 1992; Henneberg et al., 1993; Henneberg and Kaschka, 1997). Otherwise, there is a number of immunological results in the literature of which the significance and specificity
for schizophrenic diseases cannot as yet be finally appraised, e.g. the
description of atypical lymphocytes (Lahdelma et al., 1995).

Future interest will be focused on the specificity of the humoral and
cellular immune phenomena observed, the exact characterization of the
reaction partners involved and the search for disease-specific mechanisms.

To summarize, meticulous analysis of individual cases and diagnostic or genetic subgroups which have been defined especially carefully is
required in order to disclose complex etiopathogenetic patterns. These
may comprise disorders at various cybernetically interlinked levels.

Conclusions

In the meantime, there is no longer any doubt as to the existence
of bidirectional interactions between the central nervous system and

the immune system. The future task will be to characterize them more precisely and to show what levels of integration of the central nervous system (e.g. pituitary gland, hypothalamus or superordinate structures) are involved in these interactions.

Moreover, it will be important to identify and characterize possible factors interfering with these bidirectional interactions. In particular, infectious agents such as conventional viruses or unconventional agents as well as autoantibodies against relevant CNS antigens are likely to play a role. Precise knowledge of such factors is the essential prerequisite for the development of specifically targeted strategies of treatment. Systems for classifying psychiatric diseases are still not entirely satisfactory. It therefore appears conceivable to use immunological parameters to differentiate subtypes in schizophrenia or affective disorders along the lines of a biological-functional classification.

References

Ader R, Cohen N (1982) Behaviourally conditioned immunosuppression and murine systemic lupus erythematosus. Science 215:1534–1536

Ader R, Felten DL, Cohen N (1991) Psychoneuroimmunology, 2nd ed. Academic Press, San Diego

Baillarger L (1857) Example de contagion d'un délire monomanique. Monit Hosp 45:19–35

Besedovsky HO, del Rey A, Sorkin E (1981) Lymphokines containing supernatants from Con A-stimulated cells increase corticosterone blood levels. J Immunol 126: 385–387

Besedovsky HO, del Rey A, Sorkin E (1985) Immunological-neuroendocrine feedback circuits. In: Guillemin R, Cohn M, Melnechuk T (eds) Neural modulation of immunity. Raven Press, New York, pp 165–177

Besedovsky HO, del Rey A, Sorkin E, Dinarello C (1986) Immunoregulatory feedback between interleukin-1 and gluco-corticoid hormones. Science 233:652–654

Bogendörfer L (1927) Über den Einfluß des Zentralnervensystems auf Immunitätsvorgänge. Arch Exp Pathol Pharmakol 124:65–72

Brown SL, Blalock JE (1991) Recombinant interleukin-6 stimulation of pituitary ACTH secretion requires interleukin-1. In: Racagni G, Brunello N, Fukuda T (eds) Biological psychiatry, vol 2. Excerpta medica, Amsterdam, pp 115–121

Bulloch K (1985) Neuroanatomy of lymphoid tissue: a review. In: Guillemin R, Cohn M, Melnechuk T (eds) Neural modulation of immunity. Raven Press, New York, pp 111–141

Carrier M, Russell DH, Wild JC, Emery RW, Copeland JG (1987) Prolactin as a marker of rejection in human heart transplantation. J Heart Transplant 6:290–292

Cassileth BR, Lusk EJ, Miller DS, Brown LL, Miller C (1985) Psychosocial correlates of survival in advanced malignant disease? N Engl J Med 312:1551–1555

Cervera-Enguix S, Rodriguez-Rosado A (1994) Depression and monocyte dysfunction: a follow-up study. Eur Psychiatry 9:293–298

Chengappa KNR, Ganguli R, Yang ZW, Shurin G, Brar JS, Rabin BS (1995) Impaired mitogen (PHA) responsiveness and increased autoantibodies in Caucasian schizophrenic patients with HLA B8/DR3 phenotype. Biol Psychiatry 37:546–549

Galinowski A, Barbouche R, Truffinet P, Louzir H, Poirier MF, Bouvet O, Loo H, Avrameas S (1992) Natural autoantibodies in schizophrenia. Acta Psychiatr Scand 85:240–242

Ganguli R, Brar JS, Solomon W, Chengappa KNR, Rabin BS (1992) Altered interleukin-2 production in schizophrenia: association between clinical state and autoantibody production. Psychiatry Res 44:113–123

Gatti G, Angeli A, Carignola R (1992) Chronobiology of endocrine-immune interactions. In: Touitou A, Haus E (eds) Biologic rhythms in clinical and laboratory medicine. Springer, Berlin Heidelberg New York Tokyo, pp 363–374

Goodkin K, Mulder DL, Blaney NT, Ironson G, Kumar M, Fletcher MA (1994) Psychoneuroimmunology and human immunodeficiency virus type 1 infection revisited. Arch Gen Psychiatry 51:246–248

Henneberg AE, Ruffert S, Henneberg H-J, Kornhuber HH (1993) Antibodies to brain tissue in sera of schizophrenic patients – preliminary findings. Eur Arch Psychiatry Clin Neurosci 242:314–317

Henneberg AE, Kaschka WP (eds) (1997) Immunological alterations in psychiatric diseases. Karger, Basle (Adv Biol Psychiatry 18)

Hofbauer B (1846) Infectio psychica. Österr Med Wochenschr 39:1183–1188

Husband AJ (1993) Psychoimmunology. CNS-immune interactions. CRC Press, Boca Raton Ann Arbor London Tokyo

Irwin M, Brown M, Patterson TL, Hauger RL, Quayhagen M, Quayhagen M, Grant I (1991) Catecholamines, neuro-peptide Y and immune function in Alzheimer caregiver stress. In: Racagni G, Brunello M, Fukuda T (eds) Biological psychiatry, vol 2. Excerpta medica, Amsterdam, pp 567–569

Kaschka WP (1984) Die Psychopathologie der Multiplen Sklerose. Nervenheilkunde 3:72–77

Kaschka WP (1985) Klinisch-immunologische Untersuchungen bei neuropsychiatrischen Erkrankungen. Ein Beitrag zur Immunpathologie der Multiplen Sklerose, der Myasthenia gravis und der endogenen Psychosen. Thieme, Stuttgart

Kaschka WP (1989) Die Virushypothese der endogenen Psychosen – aktueller Stand der Forschung. In: Saletu B (ed) Biologische Psychiatrie. Thieme, Stuttgart New York, pp 137–142

Kaschka WP (1995) Immunologische und virologische Forschungsansätze in der Psychiatrie. In: Lieb K, Riemann J, Berger U (eds) Biologisch-psychiatrische Forschung. G Fischer, Stuttgart, pp 145–166

Kaschka WP, Aschauer HN (Eds.) (1990) Psychoimmunologie. Thieme, Stuttgart New York

Lahdelma RL, Katila H, Hirata-Hibi M, Andersson L, Appelberg B, Rimón R (1995) Atypical lymphocytes in schizophrenia. Eur Psychiatry 10:92–96

Lishman WA (1987) Organic psychiatry. The psychological consequences of cerebral disorder, 2nd ed. Blackwell, Oxford

Maes M (1994) Cytokines in major depression. Biol Psychiatry 36:498–499

Maes M, Wauters A, Neels H, Scharpé S, Van Gastel A, D'Hondt P, Peeters D, Cosyus P, Desnyder R (1995a) Total serum protein and serum protein fractions in depression: relationships to depressive symptoms and glucocorticoid activity. J Affect Disord 34:61–69

Maes M, Bosmans E, Meltzer HY (1995b) Immunoendocrine aspects of major depression. Relationships between plasma interleukin-6 and soluble interleukin-2 receptor, prolactin and cortisol. Eur Arch Psychiatry Clin Neurosci 245:172–178

McAllister CG, Rapaport MH, Pickar D, Paul SM (1991) Autoimmunity and schizophrenia. In: Tamminga CA, Schulz SC (eds) Advances in neuropsychiatry and psychopharmacology, vol 1. Schizophrenia research. Raven Press, New York, pp 111–118

McDaniel, JS (1992) Psychoimmunology: implications for future research. Southern Med J 85:388–402

Müller N, Hofschuster E, Ackenheil M, Eckstein R (1993) T-cells and psychopathology in schizophrenia: relationship to the outcome of neuroleptic therapy. Acta Psychiatr Scand 87:66–71

Perry S, Fishman B, Jacobsberg L, Frances A (1992) Relationships over 1 year between lymphocyte subsets and psychosocial variables among adults with infection by human immunodeficiency virus. Arch Gen Psychiatry 49:396–401

Piesiur-Strehlow B, Poser S, Felgenhauer K (1988) Paranoid-halluzinatorische Psychose als Manifestation einer Multiplen Sklerose. Nervenarzt 59:621–623

Rabkin JG, Wiliams JBW, Remien RH, Goetz RR, Kertzner R, Gorman JM (1991) Depression, lymphocyte subsets, and human immunodeficiency virus symptoms on two occasions in HIV-positive homosexual men. Arch Gen Psychiatry 48:111–119

Rapaport MH (1994) Immune parameters in euthymic bipolar patients and normal volunteers. J Affect Disord 32:149–156

Rapaport MH, Lohr JB (1994) Serum-soluble interleukin-2 receptors in neuroleptic-naive schizophrenic subjects and in medicated schizophrenic subjects with and without tardive dyskinesia. Acta Psychiatr Scand 90:311–315

Saphier D, Ovadia H (1990) Elektrophysiologische Parameter im Gehirn bei Immunreaktionen. In: Kaschka WP, Aschauer HN (eds) Psychoimmunologie. Thieme, Stuttgart New York, pp 25–31

Schiffer RB, Hoffman SA (1991) Behavioral sequelae of autoimmune disease. In: Ader R, Felten DL, Cohen N (eds) Psychoneuroimmunology, 2nd ed. Academic Press, San Diego, pp 1037–1066

Schott K, Batra A, Klein R, Bartels M, Koch W, Berg PA (1992) Antibodies against serotonin and gangliosides in schizophrenia and major depressive disorder. Eur Psychiatry 7:209–212

Sperner-Unterweger B, Barnas C, Fuchs D, Kemmler G, Wachter H, Hinterhuber H, Fleischhacker WW (1992) Neopterin production in acute schizophrenic patients: an indicator of alterations of cell-mediated immunity. Psychiat Res 42:121–128

Stein M, Trestman RL (1990) Psychiatric perspectives of brain, behavior, and the immune system. In: Waksman BH (ed) Immunologic mechanisms in neurologic and psychiatric disease. Raven Press, New York, pp 166–169

Stein M et al. (1985) Bereavement, depression, stress, and immunity. In: Guillemin R, Cohn M, Melnechuk T (eds) Neural modulation of immunity. Raven Press, New York, pp 29–44

Stites DP (1987) Clinical and laboratory methods for detection of cellular immune function. In: Stites DP, Stobo JD, Wells JV (eds) Basic and clinical immunology, 6th ed. Appleton and Lange, Norwalk Los Altos, pp 285–303

Taller AM, Asher DM, Pomeroy KL, Eldadah BA, Godec MS, Falkai PG, Bogerts B, Kleinman JE, Stevens JR, Fuller Torrey E (1996) Search for viral nucleic acid sequences in brain tissues of patients with schizophrenia using nested polymerase chain reaction. Arch Gen Psychiatry 53:32–40

Wollenberg R (1889) Über psychische Infektion. Arch Pychiatrie 20:62-88

Wybran J (1985) Enkephalins, endorphins, substance P, and the immune system. In: Guillemin R, Cohn M, Melnechuk T (eds) Neural modulation of immunity. Raven Press, New York, pp 157–161

Correspondence: Prof. Dr. W. P. Kaschka, Abteilung Psychiatrie I, Universität Ulm und Zentrum für Psychiatrie Weissenau, Ravensburg-Weissenau, Weingartshofer Strasse 2, Postfach 20 44, D-88190 Ravensburg, Federal Republic of Germany.

The role of the autonomous nervous system in the dialogue between the brain and immune system

K. Schauenstein[1], I. Rinner[1], P. Felsner[1], P. Liebmann[1], H. S. Haas[1], D. Hofer[1], A. Wölfler[1], and W. Korsatko[2]

[1] Department of General and Experimental Pathology, and
[2] Department of Pharmaceutical Chemistry, University of Graz, Austria

Introduction

The concept of an extrinsic regulation of the immune system through neuroendocrine signals is well established, as is the fact that the immune system in turn informs the brain about contacts with antigens via "immunotransmitters", i.e. cytokines and/or hormones with central effects [1]. All these data that have accumulated during the last twenty years have contributed to the vision of the immune system as "the sixth sense" [2]. While there is certainly still more work needed to define the physiology of this concept in all details, strong evidence has been obtained that the immune-neuroendocrine dialogue is of relevance for the homeostasis of the immune response, as defects in the activation of the hypothalamo-pituitary-adrenal (HPA) axis by immune signals were found to be associated with and/or to predispose to spontaneously occurring [3] and experimentally induced autoimmune diseases in animal models [4, 5], and there is evidence that the same is true also in humans [6]. A large body of more recent literature data strongly suggests that this dialogue involves not only the hypothalamus, but several other brain areas, notably the structures of the "Limbic System" (for review see [7]).

Neuroendocrine immunoregulation in vivo becomes obvious under conditions that elicit somatic stress responses. This has been documented in numerous clinical and experimental studies, in which the effects of physical or psychological stressors on immune functions have been examined [8]. However, the results reported are contradictory and depend on animal species, quantity and/or quality of the stressor applied, and immune function investigated. In one of our earlier studies in the rat model we could show that in one and the same individual different doses of a stressor can have opposite effects on immune functions, and that the reactivity of lymphocytes in different compartments of the immune system is differently regulated by neuroendocrine signals [9]. Another parameter that obviously determines the sensitivity of immune functions towards neuroendocrine influences lies in the complexity of the immune response. This is reflected by the well known regulatory dependence on its kinetics, where the phase of sensitization and initiation is generally by far more prone to regulatory influence, as compared to the effector phase. Furthermore, it is to be expected that the quantity and/or quality of an immune response determines the resistance against neuroendocrine signals. This notion was confirmed by observations by us suggesting that spontaneous or experimentally elicited autoimmune responses are by far more sensitive to stress effects as compared to the vigorous response against heteroantigens [3, 10].

Thus, it can be summarized that somatic stress responses do significantly influence immune functions in vivo, whereby the actual outcome in a given individual is not always predictable and depends on various parameters of both the specific stressor and the specific immune response under investigation. Similarly, the "talking back" of the immune system to the brain is expected to be equally complex and quantitatively determined by several parameters that still remain to be defined.

In the following we will review our data in the rat model on the in vivo role of the autonomous nervous system in this context, which were performed to examine if and how disturbances in the adrenergic/cholinergic balance may affect the immune-neuroendocrine interplay, and to better understand functional relationships between the immune and the adrenergic and cholinergic systems.

Adrenergic immunoregulation and the role of melatonin

Beginning with the early seventies a vast literature on morphological and functional interrelationships between the sympathetic nervous system and the immune system has accumulated. Lymphoid organs are strongly innervated by adrenergic fibres, the terminals of which come in close "synapsis like" apposition with lymphoid cells [11]. Furthermore, lymphocytes express β-adrenergic receptors in dependence of lineage and activation stage [12], the presence of α-adrenergic receptors by radioligand binding has been documented for human lymphocytes only [13]. Concerning adrenergic effects on immune functions the data are numerous and conflicting. Both enhancement and suppression of lymphocyte functions have been ascribed to either α- or β-adrenergic mechanisms, which may be due to reasons of complexity as outlined in the previous section, but also to differences in the experimental approach, particularly between in vivo and in vitro studies.

The aim of our own studies was to define in vivo effects of chronically (20 hours) increased levels of peripheral catecholamines, such as adrenalin and noradrenalin, on lymphocyte functions in the rat model. The experimental approach consists in the s. c. implantation of retard tablets that continuously release defined amounts of adrenergic agonists or antagonists into circulation [14]. This technology avoids handling stress effects (see previous section) due to repeated injections that may interfere with effects of the adrenergic treatment proper. The data obtained with this system [15] are summarized as follows: (i) a 20 hours treatment with catecholamines had no (adrenalin) or only a marginal (noradrenalin) suppressive effect on the ex vivo proliferative response of peripheral blood lymphocytes (PBL) to Concanavalin A, (ii) combination of either catecholamine with propranolol, or other β-blockers, resulted in profound suppression of this T cell responsiveness, whereas concomittant α-blockade with phentolamine had no effect, neither had β- or α-blockade per se a measurable effect, (iii) in contrast to PBL, spleen cells were consistently resistant to chronic α-adrenergic treatment.

In the following we have shown that this α-mediated suppression of lymphocyte activation does not represent a general stress symptom due to metabolic waste, nor is it due to secondarily elicited glucocorticoids, or to quantitative shifts in total T cells ($CD3^+$) or $CD4^+/CD8^+$ subsets in PBL. More recently, we could confirm this effect with the synthetic α_2-agonist clonidine, which, again only in combination with β-blockade, led to significant suppression of T cell proliferation [16], whereas methoxamine (α_1) or isoproterenol (β) had no effect. Furthermore, we observed an analogous suppressive effect on the proliferative T-cell response one hour after a single i. p. injection of the indirect sympathomimetic drug tyramine in combination with β-blockade. Thus, this phenomenon is not an artefact inherent to treatment with exogenous catecholamines, but is likewise observed under enhanced release of endogenous NA from peripheral terminals. Interestingly, the effect of tyramine was again restricted to PBL, leaving the mitogenic reactivity of splenic T-lymphocytes unaffected, which in view of the aforementioned intense sympathetic innervation of the spleen seems puzzling and is presently further investigated [16].

These data were in agreement with earlier studies of Besedovsky et al. [17] and contradicted, at least in the rat model, the significance of a β-adrenergic immunosuppression in vivo. They also suggested that a significant adrenergic in vivo effect on immune functions requires not only enhanced levels of agonists, but also an alteration in the α/β receptivity. Very recently we obtained strong evidence in the same model that the pituitary hormone melatonin plays an important and physiological role to protect the reactivity of lymphocytes from α-adrenergic inhibition. This was concluded from the following set of data, as schematically depicted in Fig. 1: (i) Substitution of animals with pharmacological doses of melatonin strongly counteracted the suppression of PBL responsiveness induced by the combination of noradrenaline and propranolol, and (ii) inhibition of the endogenous melatonin production by exposing the animals to a 24 hours constant light cycle enhanced the suppressive effect of α-adrenergic treatment similarly to what was observed with β-blockade [18].

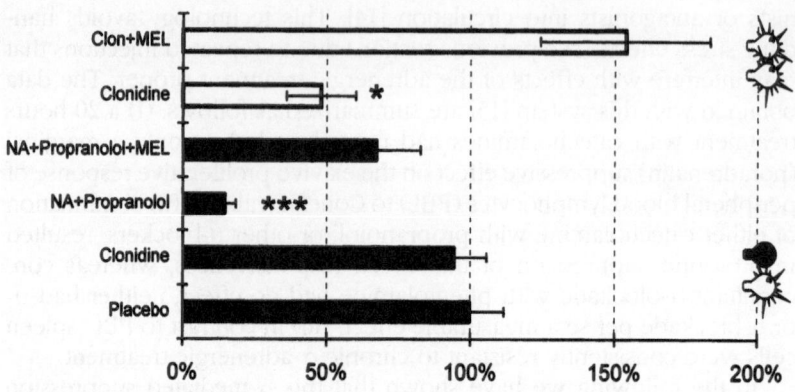

Fig. 1. Melatonin (MEL) protects lymphocytes from chronic α-adrenergic stress. The suppressive effect of retard tablets containing noradrenalin (NA) and propranolol is inhibited by oral administration of MEL (NA + propranolol + MEL). Functional pinealectomy (light/light cycle) leads to suppression by α_2-agonist clonidine, which at light/dark cycle has no effect. The suppression is again counteracted by MEL (Clon + MEL)

Accordingly it appears that the pharmacological β-blockade renders rat PBL susceptible against noradrenergic stimuli by inhibiting the release of melatonin from the pituitary gland, which supposedly exerts immunoprotective effects against stress influences (for review see [19]). Experiments are presently underway to examine, if or to what extent this concept is valid in humans.

The immune system as part of the cholinergic system?

Much less was known until recently about cholinergic-immune system interrelationships. The thymus has been reported to be innervated by cholinergic fibres [20], which, however, was questioned by other authors [21]. Concerning the spleen there is no evidence of cholinergic innervation, although low activities of both acetylcholine (ACh) and its synthetic enzyme choline acetyltransferase (ChAT) have been detected in the spleen of several species [22]. Human and rodent lymphocytes from thymus, spleen and peripheral blood were reported to express muscarinic and nicotinic cholinergic receptors [23], as well as a cellular acetylcholine esterase (AChE) [24]. Finally, cholinergic agents were reported to influence immune functions in vivo and in vitro [25, 26, 27], although the physiological source of the specific ligand, i.e. acetylcholine, in immune organs remained obscure.

In our own studies to investigate chronic cholinergic stimulation in the rat model using a similar technology as described for the adrenergic treatment we obtained evidence that the cholinergic system is intrinsically involved in the immuno-neuroendocrine dialogue [28]. This was concluded from the following data: (i) Altering the endogenous cholinergic tonus by treatment with the AChE inhibitor physostigmine or the muscarinic antagonist atropine influenced lymphocyte functions of different compartments in different ways, suggesting an enhancing cholinergic effect on lymphocytes from thymus and spleen, but not in PBL, (ii) chronic physostigmine treatment prior to immunization with antigen was found to abrogate the activation of the HPA axis due to immunization, and (iii) three days after immunization with antigen a transient increase in affinity and decreased numbers of muscarinic receptors in the gyrus hippocampus was observed. In another study we could show that acetylcholine via a nicotinergic effect on thymic epithelial cells inhibits apoptosis and thereby may affect the maturation of thymic lymphocytes [29].

Finally, we obtained evidence that lymphocytes not only react to, but also produce the neurotransmitter acetylcholine. Using a radioenzymatic method [30] we were able to detect the synthesis of acetylcholine in homogenates of isolated rat lymphocytes from thymus, spleen and peripheral blood, as well as in several murine and human lymphoid cell lines [31]. The activity of ChAT found in rat thymus lymphocytes was quantitatively very similar to what has been reported elsewhere with murine thymus tissue homogenates [32], and we concluded that this activity may have been entirely due to lymphocyte derived ChAT, rather than to cholinergic innervation. In very recent studies using a set of four different primers we detected the ChAT mRNA message in thymic and peripheral rat lymphocytes by means of RT PCR techniques (Fig. 2), and showed that the synthesis and release of acetylcholine are increased in polyclonally activated cells [33, 34].

Conclusions

The experimental results reviewed herein confirm that both the adrenergic and cholinergic autonomous nervous systems take part in the immune-neuroendocrine network. As it emerges from these data, the integration of the immune system with the parasympathetic nervous system may be much closer and more direct than the one with the adrenergic system. Cholinergic in vivo stimulation was found to directly interfere with the activation of the HPA axis due to immunization, which may facilitate unwanted immune responses, no such effect was found under adrenergic treatment (Felsner et al., unpublished observations). Acetylcholine was found to influence survival and differentiation of thymic lymphocytes, whereas catecholamines had no effect (Rinner et al., unpublished), and finally, immune cells were found not only to

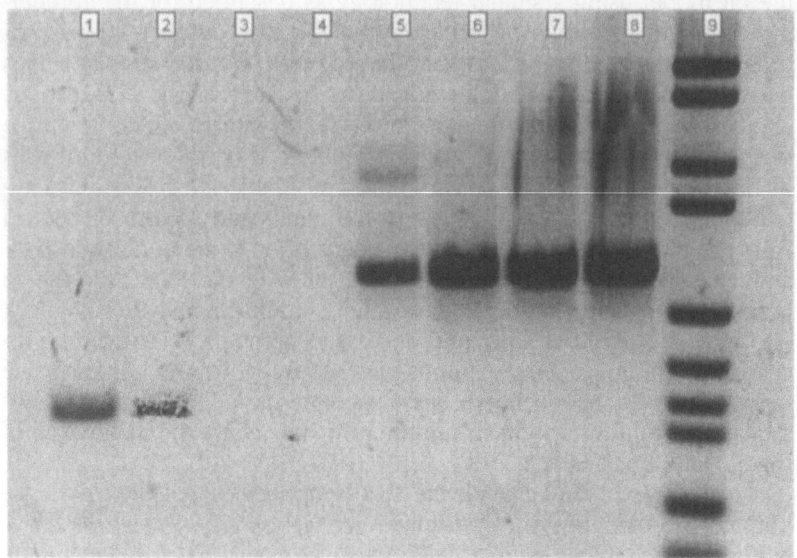

Fig. 2. Detection of mRNA for Choline-acetyltransferase (ChAT) by means of Reverse Transcriptase Polymerase Chain Reaction (RT-PCR). Lanes 1 and 2 show the PCR DNA product obtained with a primer pair specific for the coding part of the ChAT gene, derived from mRNA of PBL (1) and spinal cord (2). No signal is detected in liver (3) and heart (4). Lanes 5–8 show the expression of a control gene (β-actin) in PBL, spinal cord, liver, heart. Lane 9 = molecular weight standard

express functional cholinergic receptors and acetylcholine esterase, but also to be equipped to synthesize the specific ligand to these surface molecules, i.e. acetylcholine, which may be instrumental to communication with the autonomous nervous system, as well as contribute to autocrine immunoregulatory mechanisms. Even though we [32] and others [35] have found also catecholamines in rat and human lymphocytes, attempts to detect the mRNA expression of synthesizing enzymes, i.e. tyrosine hydroxylase and dopamin β-hydroxylase, were unsuccessful (Rinner et al., unpublished).

Further studies are underway to investigate the mechanisms by which immune cells release acetylcholine and to better define the possible physiological role(s) of lymphocyte derived neurotransmitters in the regulation of the immune system and its dialogue with the central nervous system.

Acknowledgements

The experiments reviewed herein were supported by the Austrian Science Foundation (projects 7509, 7038, 9925, 11130) and by the "Jubiläumsfonds der Österreichischen Nationalbank" (projects 3556 and 4349).

References

[1] Cotman CW, Brinton RE, Galaburda A, McEwen B, Schneider D (1987) The neuro-immune-endocrine connection. Raven Press, New York

[2] Blalock JE (1994) The immune system – our sixth sense. The Immunologist 2: 8–15

[3] Schauenstein K, Faessler R, Dietrich H, Schwarz S, Kroemer G, Wick G (1987) Disturbed immune-endocrine communication in autoimmune disease. Lack of corticosterone response to immune signals in obese strain chickens with spontaneous autoimmune thyroiditis. J Immunol 139:1830–1833

[4] Sternberg EM, Hill JM, Chrousos GP, Kamilaris T, Listwak SJ, Gold PW, Wilder RL (1989) Inflammatory mediator-induced hypothalamic-pituitary-adrenal axis activation is defective in streptococcal cell wall arthritis-susceptible Lewis rats. Proc Natl Acad Sci USA 86:4771–4775

[5] Mason D, MacPhee I, Antoni F (1990) The role of the neuroendocrine system in determining genetic susceptibility to experimental allergic encephalomyelitis in the rat. Immunology 70:1–5

[6] Berczi I, Baragar FD, Chalmers IM, Keystone EC, Nagy E, Warrington RJ (1993) Hormones in self tolerance and autoimmunity: a role in pathogenesis of rheumatoid arthritis? Autoimmunity 16:45–56

[7] Haas HS, Schauenstein K (1997) Neuroimmunomodulation via limbic structures – the neuroanatomy of psychoimmunology. Progr Neurobiol 52:195–222

[8] Keller SE, Schleifer SJ, Demetrikopoulos MK (1991) Stress-induced changes in immune function in animals: hypothalamo-pituitary-adrenal influences. In: Ader R, Felten DL, Cohen N (eds) Psychoneuroimmunology, 2nd edn. Academic Press, New York, pp 771–787

[9] Rinner I, Schauenstein K, Mangge H, Porta S, Kvetnansky R (1992) Opposite effects of mild and severe stress on in vitro activation of rat peripheral blood lymphocytes. Brain Behav Immun 6:130–140

[10] Schauenstein K, Rinner I, Felsner P, Hofer D, Mangge H, Skreiner E, Liebmann P, Globerson A (1994) The role of the adrenergic/cholinergic balance in the immune-neuroendocrine circuit. In: Berczi I, Szelenyi J (eds) Advances in psychoneuroimmunology. Plenum Press, New York, pp 349–356

[11] Felten DL, Felten SY, Bellinger DL, Carlson SL, Ackerman KD, Madden KS, Olschowski JA, Livnat S (1987) Noradrenergic sympathetic neural interactions with the immune system: structure and function. Immunol Rev 100:225–260

[12] Khan MM, Sansoni P, Silverman ED, Engleman EG, Melmon KL (1986) Beta-adrenergic receptors on human suppressor, helper and cytolytic lymphocytes. Biochem Pharm 7:1137–1142

[13] Titinchi S, Clark B (1984) Alpha2-adrenoceptors in human lymphocytes: direct

characterization by (^{3}H) yohimbine binding. Biochem Biophys Res Commun 121:1–7

[14] Korsatko W, Porta S, Sadjak A, Supanz S (1982) Implantation von Adrenalin-retard Tabletten zur Langzeituntersuchung in Ratten. Pharmazie 37:565–568

[15] Felsner P, Hofer D, Rinner I, Mangge H, Gruber M, Korsatko W, Schauenstein K (1992) Continuous in vivo treatment with catecholamines suppresses in vitro reactivity of rat peripheral blood T-lymphocytes via a-mediated mechanisms. J Neuroimmunol 37:47–57

[16] Felsner P, Hofer D, Rinner I, Korsatko W, Schauenstein K (1995) In vivo immunosuppression by enhanced catecholamines in the rat model is due to activation of peripheral a_2-receptors. J Neuroimmunol 57:27–34

[17] Besedovsky HO, Del Rey A, Sorkin E, Da Prada M, Keller HH (1979) Immunoregulation mediated by the sympathetic nervous system. Cell Immunol 48: 346–355

[18] Liebmann P, Hofer D, Felsner P, Wölfler A, Schauenstein K (1996) Beta-blockade enhances adrenergic immunosuppression in rats via inhibition of melatonin release. J Neuroimmunol 67:137–142

[19] Liebmann P, Wölfler A, Schauenstein K (1997) Melatonin and the immune system. Int Arch Allergy Immunol 112:203–211

[20] Bulloch K (1988) A comparative study of the autonomous nervous system innervation of the thymus in the mouse and chicken. Int J Neurosci 40:129–140

[21] Nance DM, Hopkins DA, Bieger D (1987) Re-investigation of the innervation of the thymus gland in mice and rats. Brain Behav Immun 1:134–147

[22] Felten SY, Felten DL (1991) Innervation of lymphoid tissue. In: Ader R, Felten DL, Cohen N (eds) Psychoneuroimmunology, 2nd edn. Academic Press, New York, pp 27–69

[23] Maslinski W (1989) Cholinergic receptors on lymphocytes. Brain Behav Immun 3:1–14

[24] Szelenyi J, Palldi-Haris P, Hollan S (1987) Changes in the cholinergic system due to mitogenic stimulation. Immunol Lett 16:49–54

[25] Iliano G, Tell GPE, Segal MI, Cuatrecasas P (1973) Guanosine 3',5'-cyclic monophosphate and the action of insulin and acetylcholine. Proc Natl Acad Sci USA 70:2443–2447

[26] Strom TB, Sytkowski AT, Carpenter CB, Merill JB (1974) Cholinergic augmentation of lymphocyte mediated cytotoxicity. A study of the cholinergic receptor of cytotoxic T lymphocytes. Proc Natl Acad Sci USA 71:1330–1333

[27] Rossi A, Tria MA, Baschieri S, Doria G, Frasca D (1989) Cholinergic agonists selectively induce proliferative responses in the mature subpopulation of murine thymocytes. J Neurosci Res 24:369–373

[28] Rinner I, Schauenstein K (1991) The parasympathetic nervous system takes part in the immuno-neuroendocrine dialogue. J Neuroimmunol 34:165–172

[29] Rinner I, Kukulansky T, Felsner P, Skreiner E, Globerson A, Kasai M, Hirokawa K, Korsatko W, Schauenstein K (1994) Cholinergic stimulation modulates apoptosis and differentiation of murine thymocytes via a nicotinic effect on thymic epithelium. Biochem Biophys Res Comm 203:1057–1062

[30] Fonnum FA (1975) Rapid radiochemical method for the determination of choline acetyltransferase. J Neurochem 24:407–409

[31] Rinner I, Schauenstein K (1993) Detection of choline-acetytransferase activity in lymphocytes. J Neurosci Res 35:188–191

[32] Badamchian M, Damavandy H, Radojcic T, Bulloch K (1992) Choline O-acetyltransferase (ChAT) and muscarinic receptors in the Balb/C mouse thymus. Abstract, Satellite meeting of the 8th International Congress of Immunology "Advances in Psychoneuroimmunology", Budapest, August

[33] Rinner I, Felsner P, Liebmann PM, Hofer D, Wölfler A, Globerson A, Schauenstein K (1997) Adrenergic cholinergic immunomodulation in the rat model – in vivo veritas? Dev Immunol (in press)

[34] Rinner I, Kawashima K, Schauenstein K (1997) Rat lymphocytes produce and secrete acetylcholine in dependence of differentiation and activation. J Neuroimmunol (in press)

[35] Josefsson E, Bergquist J, Ekman R, Tarkowski A (1996) Catecholamines are synthesized by mouse lymphocytes and regulate function of these cells by induction of apoptosis. Immunology 88:140–146

Correspondence: Univ. Prof. Dr. K. Schauenstein, Institut für Allgemeine und Experimentelle Pathologie, Universität Graz, Mozartgasse 14, A-8010 Graz, Austria

Analysis of gene expression of human brain*

Y. Sun, R. Yolken and the **Stanley Neuropathology Consortium**

The Stanley Neurovirology Laboratory, Department of Pediatrics,
Johns Hopkins University School of Medicine, Baltimore, Md, U.S.A.

Normal cell functions are dictated by well regulated patterns of gene expression. Any insult that causes aberrant gene expression will disturb the homeostasis of a cell as a unit. Therefore, measurement of gene expression and the identification of genes that are abnormally expressed during a disease process may provide a clue to the understanding of the pathogenesis of complex human diseases which involve the interaction of genetic and environmental factors.

Schizophrenia is generally considered a disease of the human brain. However, there are no specific neuropathology changes in the brain that are consistently associated with the severity and duration of the disease. The etiology of schizophrenia is still unknown. It appears that pathogenesis of schizophrenia may involve multifactorial effect such as genetic, infectious, immunological, developmental and biochemical factors. Epidemiologic evidence on seasonality of births support the possibility of viral infection in the development of schizophrenia [1, 2]. Mechanisms of virus–host interaction are heterogeneous. At the molecular level, infectious agents can interact with hosts by interfering with its gene regulation and expression leading to functional or structural abnormalities and even death of host cells. In addition, infectious agents can trigger the activation of the host immune response which can result in the generation of cytokines and other mediators which can effect brain function. Because there is neither localized neuropathology nor specific pathologic agents recognized in association with schizophrenia, it is very difficult to take advantage of the conventional methodology of histopathology and immunology for the investigation of the role of a pathologic agent in the pathogenesis. Alternatively, recent described technology in molecular biology makes it possible to study the gene expression of cells and offers an attractive approach to the investigation of this disease.

A number of methods are available for the study of gene expression. The most widely used technique is the differential display of gene

* Research supported by the Theodore & Vada Stanley Foundation

expression from two different sources, i.e. case and control. There are many versions of differential display with characteristic advantages and disadvantages [3]. Success with this technique varies depending on the quantity and quality of the target genes. Genes that are expressed in very low amounts are not readily detected because the sensitivity of the technique is limited by visualizing a band from the gel. Polymerase chain reaction (PCR) based differential display method improves the sensitivity but at the cost of specificity. Furthermore, PCR amplification tends to favor certain size ranges of the template pool, as this technique amplifies certain DNA fragment better than the others. Although longer PCR products can be amplified with modified reaction conditions, it is difficult to adjust the PCR condition to suit all sizes in the same pool of cDNA fragments. Therefore, differential display techniques are subject to amplification bias in the relative abundance of each gene, making it difficult to quantitatively compare gene product.

Recently, a team led by Kenneth Kinzler at the Johns Hopkins University developed a new technique termed serial analysis of gene expression (SAGE) [4]. This technique allows for the evaluation of global gene expression from cells or tissue and also the comparison of the relative abundance of each gene transcripts from two or more different sources through the application of a computerized program. Briefly, messenger RNA is extracted and converted to cDNA with biotinylated oligo-dT in a standard reaction. Then, the cDNA is digested with a restriction endonuclease. Those restriction fragments of DNA with the oligo-dT are selectively collected by mixing with streptavidin coated magnetic beads in a strong magnetic field. Such fragments are then divided into equal pairs ligated to a pair of linkers respectively. Each of the linkers contains a recognition sequence for a type IIS DNA restriction enzyme which cuts the DNA at a distance 10 to 20 bp from the asymmetric recognition site. In this way, a short tag of equal length is generated for each expressed gene. Such tags are then ligated and used as templates for PCR. The sensitivity of detecting genes of low abundance is greatly increased after amplification. Because the templates are equal in size, all the PCR products produced are of the same length. Therefore, unlike the PCR of a mixed length templates, PCR bias is unlikely to occur in SAGE. The tags are then released from the linkers and ligated end-to-end by T_4 DNA ligase to form concatenate multi-tag chains. The concatenate chains are then cloned into a plasmid vector and sequenced. Clones with various lengths inserts are recorded by the number of tags and the tag sequence information, and linked to the GenBank search. By accumulating the number of tags, relative abundance of each expressed gene is obtained. Genes that are expressed aberrantly as compared to controls are considered potential candidate genes of interest. Such genes will be investigated by PCR, Northern blot hybridization and cDNA library screening.

Because of the unique efficiency of SAGE, it is possible to analyze

Table 1. Analysis of tags from 13 clones of concatemers in normal human brain

Occurrence	Number of tags	GenBank search Matched	Unmatched
4	1	0	1
3	1	1	0
2	13	4	9
1	136	38	98
Total	151	43	108

large number of RNA species in a short period of time. There are estimated 150,000 human genes. SAGE tags of 10-base would cover one million (i.e. 4^{10}) sequences of different combination. Therefore, all the expressed genes can be represented by SAGE tags. RNA species that are expressed in high abundance can be detected more readily because they accumulate more quickly than genes of low abundance. SAGE is a very attractive method for the thorough evaluation of gene expression and can be used to detect RNA species that are expressed in different amounts in different developmental stages or disease status. We have used SAGE for the analysis of RNA species expressed in human brain tissue. Our data indicate that SAGE is a potentially useful method for the analysis of RNA species in human brain. Through the analysis of only 13 clones of the concatenate tags, we were able to get sequence information of 151 tags (Table 1). Almost two-thirds (108/151) of the tags have no match in the GenBank Database. This finding suggests that most of the expressed genes in the adult human brain are still uncharacterized. All of the tags that are matched to GenBank are mRNA in nature, indicating that SAGE is specific for messenger RNA devoid of ribosomal RNA contamination (Table 2). Another important notion is that the majority of the genes are expressed in low amounts. This is not surprising given the fact that the brain is an organ of complex functions. Many more genes in the brain are still unknown and new genes in the brain are discovered continuously [5]. The one tag (AAAACATTCT) that is most frequent in this collection does not match any sequence in the GenBank. It may be a novel gene highly expressed in the brain but this needs to be proven by additional analysis. For further information on the relative abundance of these genes, more clones need to be analyzed.

The above data indicate that SAGE can be an effective method for the characterization of brain mRNA. Since SAGE relies on the binding of RNA at the 3' poly A tail, the method should be able to identify virtually all human mRNA species as well as microbial RNAs which are polyadenylated, such as those which are found in the myxovirus and paramyxovirus groups of negative-strand RNA viruses. However, in light of its general applicability SAGE has great potential for the analysis of complex human brain diseases such a schizophrenia and related disorders.

Table 2. Tag sequences matched to the GenBank

Tag sequences	n (frequency)	GenBank match
GTGGCTCACG	3 (1.8)	Human HLA class I genomic survey sequence
GATCCCAACT	2 (1.2)	Human mRNA for metallothionein from cadmium
TGATTTCACT	2 (1.2)	Human cytochrome c oxidase subunit III (COIII) pse
TGTGCTGAAC	2 (1.2)	Human transferrin mRNA, complete cds
GGGAAACCCC	2 (1.2)	Human fibroblast mRNA fragment with alu sequence
AAAATAAAGA	1 (0.6)	Human HAPI mRNA
AACCCAAAAA	1 (0.6)	Human 11kd protein mRNA
AAGCTCTCCT	1 (0.6)	Human chromogranin A mRNA
ACCCTTGGCC	1 (0.6)	H. sapiens CpG island DNA genomic Mse1 fragment
ACTTACCTGC	1 (0.6)	Human mRNA for cytochrome c oxidase subunit VIB
AGAATCGCTT	1 (0.6)	Human coatomer protein mRNA
AGGGCTTCCA	1 (0.6)	Human HepGe 3' region Mbol cDNA
AGGGTGAACG	1 (0.6)	Human synaptobrevin 2 gene
AGGTCAGGAG	1 (0.6)	Human mRNA for HLA class II DR-beta
CCAACAAGAA	1 (0.6)	Human mRNA for cell surface glycoprotein
CCACTGCACT	1 (0.6)	Hum. cortex mRNA containing an Alu repetit. elem.
CCTAGCTGGA	1 (0.6)	Human mRNA for T-cell cyclophilin
CCTGTGGTCC	1 (0.6)	Human Down Syndr. region of chromos. 21 DNA
CTTGTAATCC	1 (0.6)	Human Down Syndr. region of chromos. 21 DNA
ATGAAACCCT	1 (0.6)	Human Down Syndr. region of chromos. 21 DNA
GAACACATCC	1 (0.6)	H. sapiens mRNA for ribosomal protein L19
GACTGTGCCA	1 (0.6)	Human cytoplasmic dynein light chain 1 mRNA
GCAAGCCAAC	1 (0.6)	H. sapiens mitoch. DNA for loop attachment sequence
GGAGTGGACA	1 (0.6)	Homo sapiens ribosomal protein L18 mRNA
GGGGTAAGAA	1 (0.6)	H. sapiens phosphatidylethanolamine binding protein
GTAAGTGTAC	1 (0.6)	H. sapiens mitoch. DNA for loop attachment sequence
GTGGCACGTG	1 (0.6)	Human clone AZA1 Alu repeat sequence
GTGGCAGGTG	1 (0.6)	Human ferritin H-type chain pseudogene
GTGGCGCGCG	1 (0.6)	H. sapiens DNA for loop attachment sequence
GTTCCCTGGC	1 (0.6)	Human FAU1P pseudogene, trinucleotide repeat region
TACAAGAGGA	1 (0.6)	Human mRNA for DNA binding protein, TAXREB107
TAGGATGGGG	1 (0.6)	Human sodium/potassium-transporting ATPase beta-3
TATCCCAGAA	1 (0.6)	Human kpni repeat mRNA
TATCCTGGAA	1 (0.6)	Human AMP deaminase (AMPD3) gene, exon 6
TGCACTTCAA	1 (0.6)	H. sapiens mRNA for high endothelial venule
TGTGGGGCTC	1 (0.6)	Human mRNA for histidyl-tRNA synthetase (HRS)
TTTTACCAGT	1 (0.6)	Human chloride channel regulatory protein mRNA
TGATCTCCAA	1 (0.6)	Fatty acid synthase (human breast)
GTTTCAGGTA	1 (0.6)	Homo sapiens calcium-ATPase mRNA
GTGAAACCCT	1 (0.6)	H. sapiens mRNA for laminin
GCGAAACCCC	1 (0.6)	Human ataxia-telagiectasia locus, exon 4
AGCCACTGCG	1 (0.6)	Human coagulation factor XI gene
ACCGTGGGCT	1 (0.6)	Human creatine kinase B isoenzyme gene, exon 3

References

[1] O'Callaghan E, Gibson T, Colohan HA, Walshe D, Buckley P, Waddington JR (1991) Season of birth in schizophrenia; evidence for confinement of an excess of a winter births to patients without a family history of mental disorder. Br J Psychiatry 158:764–769

[2] Yolken RH, Torrey EF (1995) Viruses, schizophrenia and bipolar disorder (review). Clin Microbiol Rev 8:131–145

[3] Yee F, Yolken RH (1997) Identification of differentially expressed RNA transcripts in neuropsychiatric disorders. Biol Psychiatry (in press)

[4] Velculescu VE, Zhang L, Vogelstein B, Kinzler KW (1995) Serial analysis of gene expression. Science 270:484–487

[5] Adams MD, Dubnick M, Kerlavage AR, Moreno R, Kelly JM, Utterback TR, Nagle JW, Fields C, Venter JC (1992) Sequence identification of 2375 human brain genes. Nature 335:632–634

Correspondence: R. H. Yolken, M.D., Director, Stanley Neurovirology Laboratory, Pediatric Infectious Diseases, The Johns Hopkins University School of Medicine, 600 N. Wolfe Street, Blalock 1111, Baltimore, MD 21287-4933, U.S.A.

New trends in neuropsychiatry: polyimmunotherapy – a new way of treatment in neurology and psychiatry. The 5S–7S Tilz protocol and the antigen clearing deficiency syndromes

G. P. Tilz[1], U. Demel[1], G. Wieselmann[2], H. Fabisch[2], H. G. Zapotoczky[2], H. Wachter[3], and D. Fuchs[3]

[1] Clinical Immunology, University of Graz, [2] Clinic of Neuropsychiatry, LKH Graz, and [3] Department of Biochemistry, University of Innsbruck, Innsbruck, Austria

In neurology and psychiatry similar immune mechanisms play a key role as in other diseases of the body. Cellular and humoral hypersensitivity and immunodeficiency occur and may become detrimental to central and peripheral neurology as well as in psychiatry. In immunodeficiency substitution or stimulation is indicated, whereas in hypersensitivity immunosuppression is the treatment of choice. All efficient forms of treatment cause some side effects, which under special conditions may become life threatening. In order to minimise these side effects we built up a new system of "Combination Therapy" of various immunomodulating drugs which we call in analogy to the polychemotherapy "Polyimmunotherapy". This has been used for a decade of years with lower individual doses, less side effects and more therapeutical benefit.

In patients with immunodeficiency and antigen clearing deficiency syndrome, immune complexes caused by recurrent infections and reduced transport capacity of the remaining immunoglobulins are able to induce immune complex vasculitis within the CNS and PNS and within the small capillaries of the perineural tissue. All forms of neuropathology and psychiatry can result and be treated successfully by immune intervention. In patients suffering from cellular immunodeficiency stimulation has been introduced. We successfully apply gamma Interferon or the combination of GM CSF plus gamma Interferon, when phagocytic function is decreased. The protocol of application is GM CSF 200 ug followed by Gamma Interferon 0,1 ml (20 ug) the day after. Thereafter 5 g 5S gammaglobulin (Gammavenin) is used, if a clearing function of circulating antigens is required. This 5S IgG is not immunosuppressive as opposed to the 7S counterpart.

In patients suffering from low immunoglobulin levels we have been using the 5S/7S protocol for many years now, the Tilz protocol as it has been named by several researchers such as J. R. Hobbs from the Westminster Medical School. The aim is the reduction of circulating antigen overload and hence the side effects caused by the transition from antigen- to antibody-excess. Before having introduced the protocol we saw up to 9% of partially life threatening complications in the immune compromised hosts. 5S given at 5 gram-doses reduces the antigen overload without immunosuppressive properties, 7S thereafter replaces the immunoglobulin levels for the normal demand. Between 20 and 40 grams are applied according to the clinical situation and the catabolic rate of IgG calculated by us. Furthermore 7S has been used by us to suppress the phlogistic and immune response in patients with autoimmunity. Especially after plasma exchange the application of 7S is indicated in order to avoid the enhanced immune reaction with overproduction of autoantibodies after the depletion. Whether plasma exchange can be replaced by the iv application of immunoglobulins alone is a matter of debate. It does not seem to be unrealistic.

In hypersensitivity immunosuppression is necessary and the application of IVIG in the field. We use them in the case of low or subnormal IG levels in the patients. If high cellular activation is prominent ICAM 1, Neopterin, TNF are high and phlogistic reactions occur, steroids +/− Pentoxyphyllin is used. If the IL 2 axis is activated, Cy A is applied and in the case of broad activation of the immune system azathioprin or the modern Mofetil Mycophenolate is used by us. In the case of vasculitic lesions and lack of response to steroids Cyclophosphamide is used, mainly as a bolus 600 mg iv. All these immunosuppressants are used in combination if necessary.

In conclusion the new way of multi modality application of immunosuppressants the Polyimmunotherapy – as we have introduced the term – has changed the clinical picture and course of neuropathology and psychiatry.

Introduction

Immunology plays a considerable role in clinical medicine, hence in neurology and psychiatry. Increasing evidence is in favour of this strong interaction between neuro-psychiatric, endocrine, and immunologic disease. After convincing experiments and clinical observations in patients with immune complex diseases of the kidneys, skin, vessels and the brain we have introduced a systematic investigation of neuro-psychiatric and psychiatric patients and found 3 types of psychiatric immunopathologies: Immunodeficiencies with antigen clearing deficiency syndrome, auto immunity and immune complex disease related to various forms of immune complex diseases. Additionally patients with pathology in cellular activation could be observed. Having explored 200 patients with psychosis in the first attempt, about 10% of these showed immunopathology.

Material and methods

All methods used are shown in Table 1.[1] Details about the methods are standard and are given elsewhere. Briefly different types of direct and indirect immunofluorescence, nephelometry, capillary electrophoresis and subtraction capillary electrophoresis, biopsies if necessary and various types of ELISA's were used.

Therapies were carried out in accordance of the results obtained in the following ways: Auto immunity in function of signs of

- inflammation – mainly by steroids and non steroidal anti inflammatory drugs if necessary,
- cellular activation as characterised by the neopterin and TNF axis – mainly by Pentoxyfiline,
- cellular activation as characterised by the IL 2 Axis – mainly by Cy a,
- cellular activation as characterised by the CD 23 axis and/or IgE-promotion – mainly by the BRM Interferon gamma,
- polyclonal activation of the immune system – mainly by the combination with aza thioprine or the newer compound mofetil mycophenolate (which showed considerable side effects).

Immunodeficiency and antigen clearing deficiency syndrome was treated by the irreplaceable 5S/7S protocol which was named by J. R. Hobbs at the Westminster Medical School "The Tilz Protocol" and consequently carries his name. Briefly 5S Gamma globulin[2] with its short half life of 18 hours is used to reduce the phlogogenic antigenic material, to reduce the transition of the phase or zone of equivalence, thereafter the 7S is employed with the half life of 18–24 days in order to mount the prophylactic and immunoregulatory potential. Dose is dependent of the catabolic rate, which is calculated by us after various nephelometric assays to be done. In the majority of cases 5 g Gammavenin followed by 10–20 g Venimmun is sufficient in these cases exhibiting moderate immunodeficiency.

---

1 Spectrum of immunological investigations carried out at the Graz University Immunology. Additionally Neopterin has been quantified and correlated to the rest of the immune activation protocol.

2 Gammavenin, a Pepsin treated brand, is used for the 5S Immunglobuline and Venimmun for the 7S Fraction

Table 1. Synopsis of investigations carried out in patients with various disorders in neurology and psychiatry. First and second row show the profiles of auto antibodies, immune complexes and complement levels, third and fourth the immunoglobulin levels and subclasses and the cell activation markers respectively. Normal values are given in parenthesis

◇ ANF (0)	◇ Gliadin IgG (−14 U/ml)	◇ Kappa (200–440)	◇ IL2R (500–900 U/L)
◇ ds DNS (−40 U)	◇ Gliadin IgA (−14 U/ml)	◇ Lambda (110–240)	◇ Beta 2M (−2.5 mg/L)
◇ ANF Subgruppen (0)	◇ Mikrosomen (0)	◇ IgG (7–15 g/L)	◇ T8 (130–500 U/L)
	◇ Colloid (0)	◇ IgA (0,7–3,8 g/L)	◇ ICAM (130–300 ug/m)
◇ CardiolipinAk-12	◇ TG-AK (60–100 E)	◇ IgM (0,4–2,5 g/L)	◇ CD23 (2–90 U/ml)
◇ MPO (0–7/7–15 E)	◇ TPO-AK (60–100)	◇ IgE (−100 IE)	◇ TNFR (1,5–4 ug/ml)
◇ Pr3 (0–7/7–15 E)	◇ SMA (0)	◇ IgG1 (5–9 ug/ml)	◇ Weitere Untersuchungen 1
◇ BMA (0)	◇ quergestr. Musk. (0)	◇ IgG2 (1,5–5 ug/ml)	
◇ GBM (XXXE)	◇ Myocard (0)	◇ IgG3 (0,15–1 ug/ml)	◇ Weitere Untersuchungen 2
◇ Parietalz. (−10 E)	◇ Inselzellen (0)	◇ IgG4 (0,1–1,5 ug/ml)	
◇ LZM (0)	◇ Thrombozyten (0)	◇ IgA1 (1,5–2,5 ug/ml)	◇ Weitere Untersuchungen 3
◇ Bindegewebe (0)	◇ CIC C1q (−4 ug)	◇ IgA2 (0,3–0,7 ug/ml)	
◇ Mito (0)	◇ C3 (0,7–1,4 g/l)	◇ Sonstiges	◇ Weitere Untersuchungen 4

Results

With theses investigations we have been able to find abnormal immunology with the following range of order:

- Pathology in cellular activation,
- autoimmunity and polyclonal activation,
- partial immunodeficiency.

These results are the key stone for the development of new ways of therapy, what we call in analogy to polychemotherapy polyimmunotherapy for more specific immune intervention.

Whereas pathology in cellular activation can be misleading, auto immunity with polyclonal activation of the immune system and immunodeficiency induce rather specific therapeutic measurements: In auto immunity dependent of the specific immune status, steroids, azathioprine, cyclosporine a, mycophenolate mofetil and to some extent biological response modifiers such as interferon gamma[3] have been used alone or in combinations.

The irreplaceable gamma globulins are used by us for the treatment of immunodeficiencies, antigen clearing deficiency syndrome (a term coined by Tilz) and the immune modulation in hypersensitive disorders without polyclonal activation of the immune system.

With these therapies patients suffering from various psychiatric disorders with immunopathology respond well, some of them who had been dependent on psychopharmacological medications even for years behaving normally now after withdrawing them.

Discussion

Clinical immunology has become a rapidly expanding field merging in all disciplines of modern biology and of course medicine. With this credo in mind and after having observed severe psychotic manifestations on patients with immune complex vasculitis of all organs of the body such as kidneys, skin, coronary arteries, eyes, central and peripheral nervous system, we have investigated the first 200 psychotics from the out patient department of Graz University Medical School. About 10% of these showed immunopathology, differing them from the majority of the other psychotics.

Three types of immunopathology could be revealed, inducing new therapeutic procedures in the form of polyimmunotherapy.

Whereas immunotherapy consisted of steroids and azathioprine until

---

3 Imukin is used by us, giving 0,1 ml twice a week subcutaneously and checking for products of soluble cellular activation (Table 1)

some years ago, we have been able to carry out a specific immune intervention now what we call Polyimmunotherapy. The aim is to intervene more specifically according to the analysis of the disturbed immune system and to reduce the side effects to a negligible amount.

Success of our procedure is encouraging to continue our way and medical credo namely that immunology today is clinical medicine of tomorrow already now in our hands.

Correspondence: Prof. G. P. Tilz, Clinical Immunology, LKH, Auenbruggerplatz 15, A-8036 Graz, Austria.

Immunological alterations in three types of schizophrenia

H. Fabisch[1], K. Fabisch[1], H. G. Zapotoczky[1], G. P. Tilz[1],
G. Langs[1], U. Demel[2], and G. Wieselmann[1]

[1] Department of Psychiatry, and [2] Department of Clinical Immunology,
University of Graz, Austria

Immunological blood serology has been showing a manifold picture of pathological changes in patients suffering from schizophrenic disorders (DeLisi, 1986). The focus of scientific investigation has been set on zytokines and their receptors (Ganguli and Rabin, 1989; Goldstein et al., 1980; Müller et al., 1990; Villemain et al., 1989). The examination of immunoglobulins, especially antibodies against neuronal tissue (Henneberg et al., 1994), is an important part of the question, in how far immunological changes may have a causal relationship to the development of schizophrenic disorders. Another important issue concerns the search for the significance of antinuclear factors (Noy et al., 1994; O'Donnel et al., 1988; Villemain et al., 1989). Altogether the findings are rather heterogenous and there are many schizophrenic patients showing normal serological parameters.

The objective of this study is to find out if there are differences in immunological alterations between the types of acute schizophrenic disorders.

Methods

39 male inpatients with a diagnosis of paranoid (12 patients, mean age 29.6 years, SD 6.3), undifferentiated (15 patients, mean age 30.7 years, SD 6.8) or disorganized schizophrenia (12 patients, mean age 25.6 years, SD 6.3) according to DSM-IV (APA, 1994) during the acute phase of their disorder entered the study.

The immunological screening was done by using an immune serum profile (Tilz, 1993) consisting of the following parameters (normal values given in parentheses):

a) Antibodies against nuclear factors (0), DNA (max. 40 U/ml), basement membrane (max. 5 U/ml), neutrophile cytoplasm (max. 7 U/ml), and cardiolipin (max. 12 U/ml);

b) IgG (6.80–15.30 g/l), IgA (0.74–3.74 g/l), and IgM (0.40–2.48 g/l);
c) circulating immune complexes (max. 4 µEq/ml);
d) complement C3 (0.75–1.40 g/l) and C4 (0.18–0.45 g/l);
e) markers of cell activation: soluble interleukin-2 receptor (529–913 U/
   ml), beta 2-microglobulin (max. 2.4 mg/l), T8 (138–533 U/ml), intercellular adhesion molecules (129.9–297.4 µg/ml), CD 23 (2–91 U/ml),
   tumor necrosis factor receptor (1.47–4.16 ng/ml).

Serum samples examination was carried out one or two days after admission, the assessment of psychopathology was done at the same time. A quantitative assessment via the PANSS (Kay et al., 1987) was the basis for the 39 patients' DSM-IV assignment to one of the three types (paranoid type, undifferentiated type, disorganized type). The frequency of immunological alterations was compared between the three types of schizophrenia.

The statistical analysis was done by using Chi-square analysis.

Results

Table 1 shows that in the group of the 12 patients suffering from the paranoid type, only 2 had alterations of immune parameters (antibodies against basement membrane and the tumor necrosis factor were elevated). In the group of patients with the undifferentiated type there were 6 patients with pathological serological immune parameters (elevated were: antibodies against DNA, basement membrane and cardiolipin; IgA; circulating immune complexes; Il-2-R and intercellular adhesion molecules) and in the disorganized group 9 patients had pathological findings (an elevation of antibodies against nuclear factor, basement membrane, cardiolipin; IgG; circulating immune complexes; C3; Il-2-R and intercellular adhesion molecules).

Comparing the three groups concerning the frequency of immunological alterations there is only a significant difference between patients suffering from paranoid and disorganized schizophrenia, as patients with paranoid symptomatology have less alterations of their immune system (χ^2 = 6.04, df = 1, $p \leq 0.05$).

Concerning the serological immune profile there was no significant difference between the paranoid and the undifferentiated type (with its mixed symptomatology) on one side, the undifferentiated type and the disorganized type on the other. These results suggest a correlation between symptomatology and immunological alterations: the more pronounced the paranoid hallucinatory symptoms emerged as the prominent criterion the less they were accompanied by immunological alterations; a greater tendency of symptomatology to fit the disorganized type was correlated with a more pronounced immunopathology.

Table 1. Frequency of serological immunological alterations in three types of schizophrenic disorders

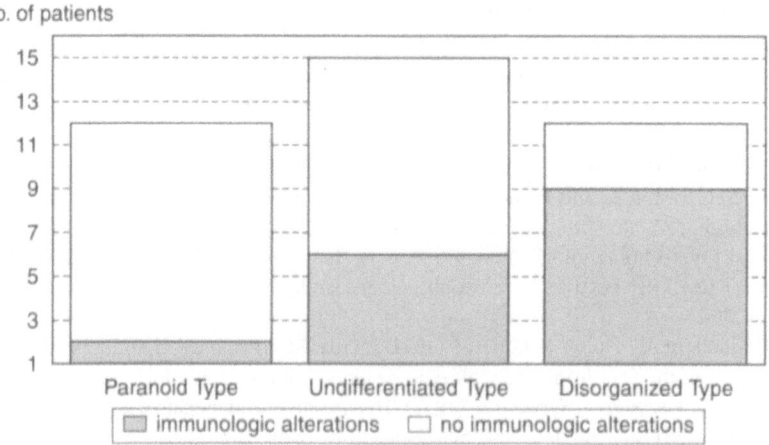

Discussion

The interpretation of immunological serological parameters raises the question in how far these alterations can be seen as the cause for psychopathology. This includes the question, if then this disorder is an endogenous psychosis or – by definition – an organic brain syndrome, which sometimes may impose as schizophrenic symptomatology (Wieselmann et al., 1995).

Further on it is remarkable that the criteria of the disorganized type (disorganized speech and behaviour, flat or inappropriate affect) are more often connected to pathological immune parameters.

The data of this study may be interpreted as follows: The pathological immune parameters may be either of etiopathogenetic importance (which is contradicted by the fact that in most cases the only use of neuroleptics – without immune suppressive medication – is sufficient), or the serological pathological parameters may be the expression of somatic vulnerability. This vulnerability may serve as a cofactor and may support the development of schizophrenic experiencing and behavior.

The authors favor the opinion that in most cases of schizophrenic disorders pathological immune parameters are not so much of etiopathogenetic influence (in the sense of an organic brain syndrome) but rather play a role as vulnerability factor.

References

American Psychiatric Association (1994) Diagnostic and statistical manual of mental disorders, 4th edn, DSM-IV. APA, Washington DC

DeLisi LE (1986) Neuroimmunology: clinical studies of schizophrenia and other psychiatric disorders. In: Nasrallah HA, Weinberger DK (eds) The neurology of schizophrenia. Elsevier, Amsterdam, pp 377–396 (Handbook of schizophrenia, vol 1)

Ganguli R, Rabin B (1989) Increased serum interleukin 2 receptor concentration in schizophrenia and brain damaged subjects. Arch Gen Psychiatry 46:292

Goldstein AL, Rossio J, Kolyaskina GL, Emory LE, Overall JE, Thurman GB, Hatcher I (1980) Immunological components in schizophrenia. In: Baxter C, Menechuk T (eds) Perspectives in schizophrenia research. Raven Press, New York, pp 249–262

Henneberg AE, Horter S, Ruffert S (1994) Increased prevalence of antibrain antibodies in the sera from schizophrenic patients. Schizophr Res 14:1–22

Kay SR, Fiszbein A, Opler LA (1987) The positive and negative syndrome scale (PANSS) for schizophrenia. Schizophr Bull 13:261–276

Müller N, Hofschuster E, Ackenheil M (1990) Zelluläres Immunsystem und Psychopathologie bei Schizophrenen. In: Kaschka WP, Aschauer HN (eds) Psychoimmunologie. Thieme, Stuttgart, pp 116–125

Noy S, Achiron A, Laor N (1994) Schizophrenia and autommunity – a possible etiological mechanism? Neuropsychobiology 30:157–159

O'Donnel M, Silove D, Wakefield D (1988) Current perspectives on immunology and psychiatry. Aust N Z J Psych 22:366–382

Tilz GP (1993) Klinische Immunbiologie und Immunhämatologie. In: Begemann H, Rastetter J (Hrsg) Klinische Hämatologie. Thieme, Stuttgart New York, pp 118–163

Villemain F, Chatenoud L, Galinowski A, Homo-Delarche F, Ginstet D, Loo H, Zarifan E (1989) Aberrant T cell-mediated immunity in untreated schizophrenic patients: deficient interleukin-2 production. Am J Psychiatry 146:609–616

Wieselmann G, Fabisch H, Tilz G, Herzog G, Fabisch K, Langs G, Zapotoczky HG (1995) "Chronische Schizophrenie" oder "Organisches Psychosyndrom"? In: Platz T, König P, Schubert H (Hrsg) Betroffen von Schizophrenie. Edition pro mente, Linz, pp 137–143

Correspondence: Dr. H. Fabisch, Department of Psychiatry, University of Graz, Auenbruggerplatz 22, A-8010 Graz, Austria.

Cytokine abnormalities in schizophrenia: a review of their pathogenic significance, with particular reference to the autoimmune hypothesis

R. Ganguli

University of Pittsburgh Medical Center,
Western Psychiatric Institute & Clinic, Pittsburgh, PA, U.S.A.

Introduction

Over the past 65 years, a variety of immunologic abnormalities have been reported in association with schizophrenia. These abnormalities have included alterations in lymphocyte subpopulations, alterations in immunoglobulin production both quantitatively and qualitatively, and altered cytokine physiology (for a review see Ganguli et al., 1994). Of these immunologic findings reported in association with schizophrenia, changes in cytokine physiology appear to be the most consistent and uncontroversial. This chapter will focus primarily on the evidence of cytokine abnormalities in a subgroup of patients, and will place these findings in the framework of the hypothesis that, for this subgroup of patients, an autoimmune process may play a pathogenetic role in their disorder. First, however, since this area of research remains mired in controversy and skepticism (DeLisi, 1996), some methodologic issues will be addressed, which pertain to the theoretical and practical aspects of study design and interpretation of results.

Biological heterogeneity in schizophrenia

Many publications reporting abnormalities found in association with schizophrenia contain a cursory nod to the notion that schizophrenia may be an etiologically heterogenous syndrome. Frequently, however, the concept of heterogeneity is lost in the presentation of results, which focus on group mean differences, and in the discussion sections which rarely speak of subgroups. The remarkable inconsistency of results which characterize much research in schizophrenia as well as the lack of significant progress towards understanding its pathophysiology(ies) may well be partly due to the reluctance of researchers to acknowledge the possibility of etiologic heterogeneity. As pointed out by Victor McKusick, the eminent geneticist, research into the etiology of clinical syndromes must take into account both pleiotropism and heterogeneity (McKusick, 1969). Pleiotropism is the phenomenon whereby a single etiology can produce a wide range of clinical syndromes. Syphilis is a good example of pleiotropism. Heterogeneity is the phenomenon whereby the same clinical syndrome may arise as a result of different etiologies. An example is provided by the mucopolysaccharidosis, in which clinically similar, but biochemically and genetically different subgroups can be positively identified. In schizophrenia research there has been some reluctance to accept heterogeneity and "split" the syndrome (Tsuang, 1995). Indeed, with regard to the autoimmune hypothesis, a willingness to accept the notion of pathophysiologic subgroups is a prerequisite, since no study has ever found immunologic abnormalities in anything more than a subgroup of patients with schizophrenia (Ganguli et al., 1995).

Clinical heterogeneity in schizophrenia

Any large group of patients with schizophrenia will contain clinically definable subgroups of patients. Some of the differences between subjects may be accounted for by variations in the severity of illness, but much of the cross-sectional variation between patients also comes from the fact that groups of schizophrenics contain individuals in different states and at different stages of the disorder. Failure to account for the specific state or stage at which patients are being studied is problematic, more so for studies of variables suspected of being involved in pathophysiology than for variables which may be etiologic. With regard to the studies of immune function, there is considerable variation between studies with regard to the state or stage of illness in which patients have been studied, and in the rigor with which this has been addressed in the study design. Many inconsistencies between studies, and the consequent skepticism (DeLisi, 1996), can most likely be attributed to obvious clinical differences between the patients studied in the different samples.

Methodologic approaches to studying autoimmune disease

Starting with the description of the autoimmune phenomena in patients with thyroid disease 40 years ago (Roitt et al., 1956; Witebsky and Rose, 1955), great strides has been made in identifying pathogenic autoimmune mechanisms in numerous previously idiopathic diseases. However, it is instructive for schizophrenia researchers that, in many instances, progress was facilitated by the willingness to split syndromes into subgroups. Type I or insulin dependent diabetes mellitus (IDDM) is a case in point. Despite the reliable demonstration of islet cell antibodies in some individuals with diabetes mellitus, the possibility that this might signify a possible autoimmune pathogenesis was rejected because most diabetics did not have such autoantibodies. A breakthrough occurred when patients were divided into those who had an early on-set, and who were insulin-dependent. It is now well accepted that the latter syndrome has an autoimmune component in its pathophysiology. In studies of immune function in schizophrenia, rarely are the majority of patients found to have immunologic abnormalities. Thus, any viable hypothesis postulating autoimmune mechanisms in the pathophysiology of schizophrenia must also postulate that this mechanism is likely to account for only a (small) proportion of cases of the disorder.

Studies of cytokine physiology in schizophrenia

In reviewing this literature care must be exercised in ensuring that the precise mechanism being studied is fully understood in terms of its pathophysiologic consequences. Studies can be grouped into those which have studied the concentrations of circulating cytokines in serum, those which have examined the capacity of cells to produce cytokines upon stimulation, and those which have measured the levels of soluble cytokine receptors in the serum. Clearly, in order to interpret the significance of any alteration in the various measures referred to above, it is crucial to consider each of the above classes of studies separately. In the following section only studies published in the past 10 years are reviewed, as there has been considerable methodologic evolution with regard to the measurement of cytokines from before that time.

Interleukin-2 has been studied extensively in several autoimmune diseases and, in several of these diseases, a decrease in the capacity of lymphocytes to produce IL-2 is associated with the development and activation of the disease process (Zier et al., 1984; Catherly et al., 1986; Eisenstein et al., 1988). In fact, in animals genetically predisposed to develop autoimmune disease, it has been shown that the capacity of their lymphocytes to produce IL-2 decreases sharply just before clinical evidence of autoimmune disease appears (Dauphinee et al., 1981). Identical twins who are discordant for IDDM have been found to also be discordant for reduced IL-2 production (Kaye et al., 1986). Reduced IL-2 production in association with schizophrenia was first reported 8 years ago, and was found in both medicated and never-medicated patients (Villemain et al., 1989; Ganguli et al., 1989). Since then several studies from different countries have replicated this findings (Table 1). In fact, all 6 studies of PHA-stimulated IL-2 production, published in peer-reviewed journals, have found that acutely ill schizophrenic patients had significantly lower IL-2 production. It is probably fair to say that decreased IL-2 production is the most reliably replicated immunologic findings in schizophrenia.

Interferon gamma (INF γ), like IL-2 is produced by the TH 1 subset of T lymphocytes. Stimulation with mitogens results in its synthesis and release, also in conjunction with IL-2. Studies have reported finding decreased PHA-stimulated INF γ production in schizophrenics (Horn-

Table 1. Studies of PHA-stimulated IL-2 production in schizophrenic patients published in peer-reviewed journals

Study	Samples	Details of results*
Villemain et al., 1989	16 never-medicated Sz**	↓IL-2 production was not correlated with mitogenic response to PHA
Ganguli et al., 1989	13 acutely ill never-medicated Sz 31 acutely ill medicated Sz 26 remitted medicated Sz 51 normal controls	↓IL-2 production only in acutely ill patients. Never-medicated patients had lowest level of IL-2 production
Ganguli et al., 1992	29 acutely ill never-medicated Sz 47 acutely ill medicated Sz 46 remitted medicated Sz 98 normal controls	↓IL-2 production only in acutely ill patients, and associated with production of circulating autoantibodies
Bessler et al., 1995	7 drug-free Sz 16 medicated Sz 19 normal controls	↓IL-2 production more pronounced in drug-free patients
Hornberg et al., 1995	17 medicated inpatient Sz 20 medicated outpatient Sz 42 blood donors	↓IL-2 production and production of INF α & γ were also lower, but only IL-2 was significant
Ganguli et al., 1995	33 never-medicated Sz 33 pair-wise matched controls	↓IL-2 production was associated with negative symptoms and earlier age at onset

* All studies reported that IL-2 production in acutely ill schizophrenics was significantly decreased as compared to controls. ** Schizophrenic patients

berg et al., 1995; Wilke et al., 1996). However, Inglot et al. (1994) found decreased INF γ production in psychotic patients only in response to Newcastle Disease Virus stimulation, not in response to PHA stimulation. Table 2 summarizes the findings of studies in this area.

Studies of circulating cytokines

There have been a few studies of circulating IL-6 and of its receptor in the serum of schizophrenics (Table 3). Of these the majority have found that IL-6 is increased in the serum of schizophrenic patients. Some studies (Ganguli et al., 1994), though not all, found that the elevation in IL-6 was correlated with the length of illness. A number of studies have also found an elevation of acute phase proteins, other than IL-6 in association with schizophrenia (Maes et al., 1995).

Table 2. Studies of stimulated INF γ production published in peer-reviewed journals

Study	Samples	Details of results*
Moises et al., 1985	19 acutely ill Sz 12 healthy medical students and hospital staff	↓INF production in schizophrenic patients, but not statistically significant
Katila et al., 1989*	13 never-medicated Sz 21 previously-medicated (all acutely ill)	↓INF production was statistically significant only for INF ↓ α
Inglot et al., 1994	32 chronic Sz 13 depressed 65 normal controls	↓INF primarily in response to NDV stimulation and correlated with negative symptoms
Hornberg et al., 1995	17 medicated inpatient Sz 20 medicated outpatient Sz 42 blood donors	Production of INF α by NDV & INF γ by PHA. Production of both was lower but did not reach statistical significance
Wilke et al., 1996	49 Sz "in and outpatients" 38 blood donors	when patients were clinically subdivided, INF γ production was significantly reduced in "paranoid" patients, but not in "residual" patients

* All studies used the whole blood technique to measure capacity for INF production except for Katilla et al., who stimulated isolated and washed lymphocytes. The latter technique consistently results in lower cytokine production and is probably less reflective of in vivo conditions

Table 3. Studies of serum interleukin-6 in schizophrenic patients published in peer-reviewed journals

Study	Samples	Details of results*
Shintani et al., 1991	90 remitted medicated Sz 90 normal controls	↑ serum IL-6, 6 patients had "aberrantly evevated" serum IL-6 levels
Ganguli et al., 1994	24 never-medicated Sz 11 acutely ill medicated Sz 69 remitted medicated Sz 110 normal controls	↑ IL-6 only in remitted patients, serum IL-6 correlated with duration of illness
Maes et al., 1995	14 acutely ill Sz 10 acutely ill manic patients 21 healthy volunteers	↑ serum IL-6 in the "combined psychotic group"

In contrast to the studies of IL-6, studies of IL-2 (Barak et al., 1995; Gattaz et al., 1992) and INF (Becker et al., 1990; Gattaz et al., 1992; Inglot et al., 1994) in the serum have not found altered levels in association with schizophrenia. These negative studies of serum IL-2 and INF are in marked contrast to the consistency with which studies of stimulated IL-2 and interferon have found differences between schizophrenic patients and controls.

Discussion

It would seem to be clear that abnormalities of IL-2 and interferon production are consistently found in a subgroup of patients with schizophrenia and that these abnormalities fluctuate with changes in the clinical state. The significance of these findings for the pathophysiology of schizophrenia remains to be established. Both of the above cytokines are produced by the TH 1 subtype of helper T lymphocytes. Thus, one might postulate that a defect in T lymphocyte physiology, perhaps specifically in the TH 1 subtype is associated with acute episodes of schizophrenia. In autoimmune disease and some chronic infectious diseases, shifts from a TH 1 type of response to a TH 2 type of response is associated with a shift away from cell-mediated immune response patterns towards antibody-mediated response patterns (Reiner and Locksley, 1995). It should be noted, however, that direct evidence of a shift from a TH 1 to a TH 2 pattern of cytokine production has not so far been documented in association with relapses of schizophrenia.

Since IL-2 acts principally in an autocrine and paracrine manner it is not surprising that the changes in T lymphocyte physiology are not necessarily accompanied by changes in the circulating levels of IL-2. In fact, changes in circulating levels of IL-2 have been of little interest in the study of autoimmune disease in general. On the other hand there is some considerable evidence for "hormone-like" effects of IL-6 (Zaleman et al., 1994) and changes in the serum level of this cytokine have been extensively documented in association with schizophrenia.

Cross-sectional studies provide little help in assigning any causal direction to the associations between cytokine abnormalities and schizophrenia. The plausibility of cytokine alterations might be strengthened by the observation that the changes in IL-2 production were correlated with levels of antibody against brain peptides derived from the hippocampus, in at least one study (Yang et al., 1994). This latter finding is one of the few published studies in which a functional peripheral immune parameter has been shown to correlate with a putative mechanism for the immune system to interact with the brain.

Longitudinal studies of immune function with parallel measurement of clinical changes are ideally suited to reveal the temporal relationship between changes in immune parameters and changes in clinical state in the same patient. Thus, longitudinal studies of this design offer the best method for evaluating whether immune changes play a causal role in schizophrenia. Unfortunately, only one such study seems to be underway (Ganguli et al., 1995). Preliminary evidence from that study did provide support for the hypothesis that changes in the capacity of the patient's lymphocytes to produce IL-2 did precede the onset of psychotic symptoms, in a manner reminiscent of the decrease in IL-2 production capacity which has been documented to precede the onset of autoimmune disease in animals (Dauphinee et al., 1981).

Conclusions

It seems fairly clear that abnormalities of cytokine production can be found in subgroups of schizophrenic patients. The abnormalities appear to be restricted to decreased capacity of lymphocytes from schizophrenic patients to produce IL-2 and INF γ and increased circulating levels of IL-6. A close examination of the results show that these abnormalities have been consistently found in subgroups of patients diagnosed as schizophrenic. Taken together these findings support the plausibility of the hypothesis that this subgroup of patients may have an autoimmune component to their disorder. However, plausibility does not provide proof, nor does it provide a mechanism to explain how such immunologic abnormalities might alter brain functions in order to contribute to the development of schizophrenia.

There is considerable evidence that IL-2 receptors are present in the brain (Araujo et al., 1989; Lapchak, 1992) as well as evidence that peripherally produced IL-2 can traverse the blood brain barrier and cause changes in the central nervous system (Saris et al., 1988). Several studies have also shown that infused IL-2 has behavioral effects (Denicoff et al., 1987; Ellison et al., 1990; Nemni et al., 1992) and that it may have neuromodulatory and neurotropic functions (Nistico and DeSarro, 1991; Plata-Salaman, 1991; Hama et al., 1991; Norris, 1993; Hanisch et al., 1993; Zalcman et al., 1994). Thus it is quite plausible that alterations in IL-2 production could result in changes in the function of the CNS (Smith, 1991, 1992) or that changes observed in circulating lymphocytes might reflect abnormalities of intracerebrally-produced cytokines (Frei et al., 1989; Benvemoste, 1992). It is however, still possible that the observed changes in IL-2 production might be the result of altered brain function, since brain lesion studies in animals have been shown to result in changes in peripheral cytokine production (Nance, 1987).

Further studies could proceed in several directions. Longitudinal studies are the best means to determine the temporal sequence of immunologic changes relative to clinical changes, and also one of the best ways to assign a causal direction. Yet most studies continue to be based on cross-sectional designs. A number of studies in the literature have had small heterogenous samples and thus have been subject to a high risk of type II error. Careful attention to issues of state and stage of illness would help to increase the confidence in both positive and negative findings. Many studies have also used controls who happen to be conveniently available, but not comparable to schizophrenic patients. Since we have data indicating that factors such as race can influence cytokine production (Ganguli and Rabin, 1989), great care should be taken in the selection of control groups to ensure they are as closely matched to the patients as possible.

Clearly the role of immune abnormalities in schizophrenia needs to be pursued further. However, careful attention to methodology, sample size, and to a longitudinal approach should help to resolve many of the enduring controversies in this area of research into the pathophysiology of schizophrenia.

References

Araujo DM, Lapchak PA, Collier B, Quirrion R (1989) Localization of interleukin-2 immunoreactivity and interleukin-2 receptors in the rat brain: interaction with the cholinergic system. Brain Res 498:257–266

Barak V, Barak Y, Levine J, Nisman B, Roisman (1995) Changes in interleukin-1 beta and soluble interleukin-2 receptor levels in CSF and serum of schizophrenic patients. J Basic Clin Physiol Pharmacol 6:61–69

Becker D, Kritschmann E, Floru S, Shlomo-David Y, Gotlieb-Stematsky T (1990) Serum interferon in first psychotic attack. Br J Psychiatry 157:136–138

Benvemoste EN (1992) Inflammatory cytokines within the central nervous system: cources, function, and mechanism of action. Am J Physiol 263 (Cell Physiol 32): C1–C16

Bessler H, Levental Z, Karp L, Modai I, Djaldetti M, Weizman A (1995) Cytokine production in drug-free and neuroleptic-treated schizophrenic patients. Biol Psychiatry 38:297–302

DeLisi LE (1996) Is there a viral or immune dysfunction etiology to schizophrenia? Re-evaluation a decade later. Schizophr Res 22:1–4

Denicoff KD, Rubinoff DR, Papa MZ, Simpson C, Seipp CA, Lotze MT, Chang AE, Rosenstein D, Rosenberg SA (1987) The neuropsychiatric effects of treatment with interleukin-2 and lymphokine-activated killer cells. Ann Intern Med 107: 293–300

Ellison MD, Krieg RJ, Povlishock JT (1990) Differential central nervous responses following single and multiple recombinant interleukin-2 infusions. J Neuroimmunol 28:259–260

Frei K, Malipiero UV, Leist TP, Zinkernagel RM, Schwab ME, Fontant A (1989) On the cellular source and function of interleukin-6 produced in the central nervous system in viral diseases. Eur J Immunol 19:689–694

Ganguli R, Rabin BS (1989) Differences in interleukin-2 production in blacks and whites. N Engl J Med 320:399

Ganguli R, Rabin BS, Belle SH (1989) Decreased interleukin-2 production in schizophrenic patients. Biol Psychiatry 26:427–430

Ganguli R, Brar JS, Solomon W, Chengappa KNR, Rabin BS (1992) Altered interleukin-2 production in schizophrenia: association between clinical state and autoantibody production. Psychiatry Res 44:113–123

Ganguli R, Brar JS, Chengappa KNR, Yang ZW, Nimgaonkar VL, Rabin BS (1993) Autoimmunity in schizophrenia: a review of recent findings. Ann Med 25:489–496

Ganguli R, Yang ZW, Schurin G, Chengappa KNR, Brar JS, Gubbi AV et al. (1994) Serum interleukin-6 concentration in schizophrenia: elevation associated with duration of illness. Psychiatry Res 51:1–10.

Gattaz WF, Dalgalarrondo P, Schroder HC (1992) Abnormalities in serum concentrations of interleukin-2, interferon-alpha and interferon-gamma in schizophrenia not detected. Schizophr Res 6:237–241

Gutierrez EG, Banks WA, Kastin AJ (1993) Murine tumor necrosis factor alpha is transported from blood to brain in the mouse. J Neuroimmunol 45:137–146

Hama T, Kushima Y, Miyamoto M, Kubota M, Takei N, Hatanaka H (1991) Interleukin-6 improves the survival of mesencephalic catochelaminergic and septal cholinergic neurons from patnatal, two-week-old rats in cultures. Neuroscience 40:445–452

Hanisch UK, Seto D, Quirion R (1993) Modulation of hippocampal acetylcholine release: a potent central action of interleukin-2. J Neurosci 13:3368–3374

Hornberg M, Arolt V, Wilke I, Kruse A, Kirchner H (1995) Production of interferons and lymphokines in leukocyte cultures of patients with schizophrenia. Schizophr Res 15:237–242

Inglot AD, Leszek J, Piasecki E, Sypula A (1994) Interferon responses in schizophrenia and major depressive disorders. Biol Psychiatry 35:464–473

Katila H, Cantell K, Hirvonen S, Rimon R (1989) Production of interferon-α and -γ by leukocytes from patients with schizophrenia. Schizophr Res 2:361–365

Kaye WA, Adri MN, Soeldner JS, Rabinowe SL, Kaldany A, Kahn CR et al. (1986) Acquired deficit in interleukin-2 production in patients with type I diabetes mellitus. N Engl J Med 315:920–924

Kirch DG, Kaufmann CA, Papadopoulos NM, Martin B, Weinberger DR (1985) Abnormal cerebrospinal fluid protein indices in schizophrenia. Biol Psychiatry 20:1039–1046

Kroemer G, Andreu JL, Gonzalo JA, Martinez C (1991) Interleukin-2, autotolerance, and autoimmunity. Adv Immunol 50:147–235

Lapchak PA (1992) A role for interleukin-2 in the regulation of striatal dopaminergic function. Neuroreport 3:165–168

Licinio J, Seibyl JP, Altemus M, Charney DS, Krystal JH (1993) Elevated CSF levels of interleukin-2 in neuroleptic-free schizophrenic patients. Am J Psychiatry 150:1408–1410

Maes M, Meltzer HY, Bosmans E (1994) Immune-inflammatory markers in schizophrenia: comparison to normal controls and effects of clozapine. Acta Psychiatr Scand 89:346–351

Maes M, Bosmans E, Meltzer HY (1995) Immunoendocrine aspects of major depression. Relationships between plasma interleukin-6 and soluble interleukin-2 receptor, prolactin and cortisol. Eur Arch Psychiatry Clin Neurosci 245:172–178

McAllister CG, vanKammen DP, Rehn TJ, Miller AN, Gurklis J, Kelley ME, Yao J, Peters JL (1995) Increases in CSF levels of interleukin-2 in schizophrenia: effects of recurrance of psychosis and medication status. Am J Psychiatry 152:1291–1297

McKusick VA (1969) On lumpers and splitters, or the nosology of genetic disease. Nosology of Genetic Disease Perspectives in Biology and Medicine (Winter): 298-312

Muller N, Ackenheil M (1995) Immunoglobulin and albumin contents of cerebrospinal fluid in schizophrenic patients: the relationship to negative symptomatology. Schizophr Res 14:223–228

Muller N, Ackenheil M, Hofschuster E, Mempel W, Eckstein R (1991) Cellular immunity in schizophrenic patients before and during neuroleptic therapy. Psychiatry Res 37:147–160

Nance DM, Rayson D, Carr RI (1987) The effects of lesions in the lateral septal and hippocampal areas on the humoral immune response of adult female rats. Brain Behav Immun 1:292–305

Nemni R, Iannaccone S, Quattrini A, Smirne S, Sessa M, Lodi M, Ermino C, Canal N (1992) Effect of chronic treatment with recombinant interleukin-2 on the central nervous system of adult and old mice. Brain Res 591:248–252

Nistico G, De Sarro G (1991) Is interleukin-2 a neuromodulator in the brain? TINS 14:146–150

Norris JG, Benveniste EN (1993) Interleukin-6 production by astrocytes: induction by the neurotransmitter norepinephrine. J Neuroimmunol 45:137–146

Plata-Salaman CR (1991) Immunoregulators in the nervous system. Neurosci Behav Rev 15:185–215

Reiner SL, Locksley RM (1995) The regulation of immunity to leishmania major. Annu Rev Immunol 13:151–177

Roitt IM, Doniach D, Campbell PN, Hudson RV (1956) Autoantibodies in Hashimoto's disease. Lancet ii:820–821

Rose NR, Witebsky E (1956) Studies on organ specificity. V. Changes in the thyroid glands of rabbit following active immunization with rabbit thyroid extracts. J Immunol 76:417–427

Saris SC, Rosenberg SA, Friedman RB, Rubin JT, Barba D, Oldfield EH (1988) Penetration of recombinant interleukin-2 across the blood-cerebrospinal fluid barrier. J Neurosurg 69:29–34

Sawada M, Suzumura A, Marunouchi T (1992) TNF-alpha induces IL-6 production by astrocytes, but not by microglia. Brain Res 583:296–299

Sharief MK, Hentges R, Ciardi M, Thompson EJ (1993) In vivo relationship of interleukin-2 and soluble IL-2 receptor to blood-brain barrier impairment in patients with active multiple sclerosis. J Neurol 240:46–50

Shintani F, Kanba S, Maruo N, Nakaki T, Nibuya M, Suzuki E et al. (1991) Serum interleukin-6 in schizophrenic patients. Life Sci 49:661–664

Shintani F, Kanba S, Nakaki T, Nibuya M, Kinoshita N, Suzuki E, Yagi G, Kato R, Asai M (1993) Interleukin-1 beta augments release of norepinephrine, dopamine, and serotonin in the rat anterior hypothalamus. J Neurosci 13:3574–3581

Smith RS (1991) Is schizophrenia caused by excessive production of interleukin-2 and interleukin-2 receptors by gastrointestinal lymphocytes? Med Hypotheses 34:225–229

Smith RS (1992) A comprehensive macrophage-T-lymphocyte theory of schizophrenia. Med Hypotheses 39:248–257

Tsuang MT, Faraone SV (1995) The case for heterogeneity in the etiology of schizophrenia. Schizophr Res 17:161–175

Villemain F, Chatenoud L, Galinowski A, Homo DF, Ginestet D, Loo H et al. (1989) Aberrant T cell-mediated immunity in untreated schizophrenic patients: deficient interleukin-2 production. Am J Psychiatry 146:609–616

Wilke I, Arolt V, Rothermundt M, Weitzsch C, Homberg M, Kirchner H (1996) Investigations of cytokine production in whole blood cultures of paranoid and residual schizophrenic patients. Eur Arch Psychiatry Clin Neurosci 246:273–278

Zalcman S, Green-Johnson JM, Murray L, Nance DM, Dyck D, Anisman H, Greenberg AH (1994) Cytokine-specific central monoamine alterations induced by interleukin-1, -2 and -6. Brain Res 643:40–49

Correspondence: R. Ganguli, M.D., University of Pittsburgh Medical Center, Western Psychiatric Institute & Clinic, 3811 O'Hara Street, Pittsburgh, PA 15213-2593, U.S.A.

Relationship between immune and behavioral measures in schizophrenia

D. P. van Kammen[1,2], C. G. McAllister[1,2], and M. E. Kelley[1]

[1] Veterans Affairs Medical Center, and [2] Western Psychiatric Institute and Clinic, University of Pittsburgh, School of Medicine, Pittsburgh, PA, U.S.A.

Schizophrenia, which is a chronic but episodic disorder of unknown etiology, shares immunological features with organ specific autoimmune diseases such as multiple sclerosis (MS), rheumatoid arthritis and insulin-dependent diabetes mellitus. However, recent studies have raised the issue as to whether the reported immune disturbances in schizophrenia may be the result of a stress-induced dysregulation of CNS cytokine production, rather than a permanent immunological disorder, i.e., auto-immunity.

The Th1 subset of CD4$^+$ T lymphocytes mediate cellular immune responses, i.e., those that initiate an autoimmune-type reaction to environmental insults (e.g., prenatal viral infections or obstetric complications). In contrast, the primary mechanism of action for Th2 cells is to stimulate the production of antibodies. Differentiating between Th1 and Th2 effects can be accomplished by measuring cytokines that are representative of these two subsets of cells (e.g., Th1 cells: IL-2 and interferon γ (IFNγ); Th2 cells: interleukin 4 (IL-4), interleukin 10 (IL-10) and Transforming Growth Factor β (TGFβ)). Interleukin 6 (IL-6), originally proposed to be a Th1 cytokine, has now been shown to exhibit both Th1 and Th2 properties.

IL-2 has been primarily viewed as a immunologically relevant substance which promotes the development and maintenance of immune responses. However, IL-2 in particular, and cytokines in general, have other functions. Cytokines, including IL-1 and IL-2, have now been shown to be produced by cells within the CNS including microglia and astrocytes (Merrill, 1990). In addition, these molecules are believed to have a role in normal brain development (Merrill, 1992). Receptors for IL-2 have been demonstrated in the brain, with the highest density reported in the hippocampus (Lapchek et al., 1991), which is of interest in schizophrenia. Brown et al. (1991) have suggested that IL-2 regulates the hypothalamic-pituitary-adrenal axis, the primary mediator of stress. This raises an important issue of a possible role for the immune system in the stress mediation of relapse in schizophrenia.

Table 1. CSF immune measures and psychosis

	Haloperidol			Drug free		
	r	n	p	r	n	p
CSF IL-2	−0.001	64	ns	0.097	64	ns
CSF IL-1α	0.197	64	ns	0.056	64	ns
CSF IL-6	0.006	62	ns	0.105	60	ns
CSF TGFβ*	0.055	40	ns	−0.079	39	ns
CSF IL-10	0.350	63	0.005	0.190	62	ns

Data indicates maximum sample size for each group assay; not necessarily the same patients. * TGFβ was detected in approximately 2/3 of the sample. Psychosis measured on the 15 point Bunney–Hamburg global rating scale (Bunney and Hamburg, 1963)

Table 2. CSF immune measures and negative symptoms (total 5 global SANS items)

	Haloperidol			Drug free		
	r	n	p	r	n	p
CSF IL-2	−0.048	64	ns	0.135	64	ns
CSF IL-1α	−0.024	64	ns	0.064	64	ns
CSF IL-6	−0.046	62	ns	0.131	60	ns
CSF TGFβ*	−0.042	40	ns	0.057	39	ns
CSF IL-10	0.115	63	ns	0.351	62	0.005

Data indicates maximum sample size for each group assay; not necessarily the same patients. * TGFβ was detected in approximately 2/3 of the sample. Negative symptoms measured using the Scale for the Assessment of Negative Symptoms (SANS) (Andreasen et al., 1982)

Relapse, or the increase of symptomatology, has been the focus of our recent clinical investigations in schizophrenia (van Kammen et al., 1994, 1995, 1996). Our group has subsequently shown that the cerebrospinal fluid (CSF) levels of the cytokine interleukin-2 (IL-2), but not interleukin-1 (IL-1), were elevated in haloperidol treated patients who relapsed within 6 weeks following drug withdrawal (McAllister et al., 1995). This indicated a possible stress sensitivity in the relapsed patients which could be identified using CSF immune measures. In order to further define the role of cytokines in schizophrenic pathology, we tested for specific associations between CSF cytokine levels and behavior. Clinical studies of nonpsychiatric patients have provided support for a possible association between behavior and cytokine levels. For example, cancer patients treated with high doses of recombinant IL-2 exhibited severe behavioral and cognitive changes, including hallucinations and delusions which responded to haloperidol treatment (Denicoff et al., 1987).

The association between cytokines measured in the CSF and spe-

Table 3. CSF IL-10 in schizophrenic patients during haloperidol treatment and after haloperidol withdrawal

	Haloperidol (mean ± sd)	Drug free (mean ± sd)	N
IL-10			
Non-relapsers	5.69 ± 1.96	5.46 ± 1.95	31
Relapsers	5.64 ± 1.80	5.76 ± 1.98	31
Total group	5.66 ± 1.86	5.61 ± 1.96	62
Effect	F	df	p
Relapse	0.10	1, 60	ns
Medication	0.03	1, 60	ns
Relapse by medication	0.90	1, 60	ns

cific behavioral measures are presented in Tables 1 and 2. Data from our relapse prediction study (McAllister et al., 1995) showed no associations between CSF IL-1α or IL-2 and behavioral measures (data not published). A recent partially overlapping sample of 63 schizophrenic patients both on and off medication were evaluated for CSF IL-6, IL-10, and TGFβ. CSF IL-10 was the only measure found to correlate with psychosis or negative symptoms. Whereas psychosis was significantly associated with CSF IL-10 only on haloperidol, negative symptoms were associated with IL-10 only in the drug free state. Haloperidol withdrawal has clear effects on behavior, as evidenced by the number of patients who relapsed. However, CSF IL-10 was not effected by haloperidol withdrawal (Table 3).

We hypothesized that CSF IL-2 would be associated with psychosis due to its association with relapse in our previous report (McAllister et al., 1995). However, IL-10 was the only significant correlate found. This posed the question as to what relevance IL-10 may have to schizophrenia. It is well established that treatment with IL-2 has neuroendocrine effects, specifically on the HPA axis (Denicoff et al., 1989). Further, the HPA axis and neuroendocrine systems have been clearly linked to immune regulation (Savino and Dardenne, 1995). Specifically, it has been proposed that the HPA axis may be relevant to the regulation of the balance between Th1 and Th2 responses (Rook et al., 1994). A shift from a Th1 to a Th2 response is seen in many chronic diseases and particularly with stress. If this is the case, the increased IL-2 we found in schizophrenic patients may cause stimulation of the HPA axis, which in turn forces the system towards a Th2 response. Thus the association between higher IL-10 and higher psychosis during haloperidol treatment may indicate the system's attempt to re-stabilize itself. It has been shown that chlorpromazine, a traditional antipsychotic, up-regulates the secretion of IL-10 in vivo (Tarazona et al., 1995). In addition, pretreatment with dexamethasone, an HPA antagonist, was shown to increase IL-10 mRNA levels in vitro (Ramirez et al., 1996). If this observation also applies in vivo, the observed correlation between CSF IL-10 and psychosis may be an effect of the IL-2-based stress sensitivity we previously reported in schizophrenic patients (McAllister et al., 1995).

The significant association found between CSF IL-10 and negative symptoms in schizophrenia would seem in contrast to the finding with psychosis. However, it is clear that while some level of negative symptoms is related to psychosis, there are also "primary" or more enduring negative symptoms which do not parallel psychotic exacerbation (Carpenter et al., 1988; Tandon et al., 1995). The association with negative symptoms drug free but not on haloperidol treatment would seem to indicate that IL-10 is associated with relapse-induced negative symptoms rather than those that remain during pharmacological treatment. A similar shift to a Th2 response may be in effect with negative symptoms following drug withdrawal and relapse. One would expect, however, that the association would also pertain to psychosis, which it does not. The reason for this is unclear, but the effects of antipsychotics on IL-10 may be responsible for this discrepancy.

Clearly further research is needed investigating the immune system in response to relapse, medication, and behavior in schizophrenia. Future directions may include further explorations of the Th1/Th2 balance, and possible direct effects of the immune system on brain function in schizophrenia.

References

Andreasen NC (1982) Negative symptoms in schizophrenia: definition and reliability. Arch Gen Psychiatry 39:784–794

Brown R, Li Z, Vriend CY, Nirula R, Janz L, Falk J, Nance DM, Dyck DG, Greenberg AH (1991) Suppression of splenic macrophage interleukin-1 secretion following intracerebroventricular injection of interleukin-1β: evidence of pituitary-adrenal and sympathetic control. Cell Immunol 132:84–93

Bunney Jr WE, Hamburg DA (1963) Methods for reliable longitudinal observation of behavior. Arch Gen Psychiatry 9:280–294

Carpenter Jr WT, Heinrichs DW, Wagman AMI (1988) Deficit and nondeficit forms of schizophrenia: the concept. Am J Psychiatry 145:578–583

Denicoff KD, Rubinow DR, Papa MZ, Simpson C, Seipp CA, Lotze MT, Chang AE, Rosenstein D, Rosenberg SA (1987) The neuropsychiatric effects of treatment with interleukin-2 and lymphokine activated killer cells. Ann Intern Med 107:293–300

Denicoff KD, Durkin TM, Lotze MT, Quinlan PE, Davis CL, Listwak SJ, Rosenberg SA, Rubinow DR (1989) The neuroendocrine effects of interleukin-2 treatment. J Clin Endocrinol Metab 69:402–410

Lapchek PA, Araujo DM, Quirion R, Beaudet A (1991) Immunoautoradiographic localization of interleukin 2-like immunoreactivity and interleukin 2 receptors (Tac antigen-like immunoreactivity) in the rat brain. Neurosci 44:173–184

McAllister CG, van Kammen DP, Rehn TJ, Miller AL, Gurklis J, Kelley ME, Yao J, Peters JL (1995) Increases in CSF levels of interleukin-2 in schizophrenia: effects of recurrence of psychosis and medication status. Am J Psychiatry 152:1291–1297

Merrill JE (1990) Interleukin-2 effects in the central nervous system. Ann NY Acad Sci 594:188–199

Merrill JE (1992) Tumor necrosis factor alpha, interleukin 1 and related cytokines in brain development: normal and pathological. Dev Neurosci 14:1–10

Ramírez F, Fowell DJ, Puklavec M, Simmonds S, Mason D (1996) Glucocorticoids promote a Th2 cytokine response by CD4+ T cells in vitro. J Immunol 156: 2406–2412

Rook GAW, Hernandez-Pando R, Lightman SL (1994) Hormones, peripherally activated prohormones and regulation of the Th1/Th2 balance. Immunol Today 15: 301–303

Savino W, Dardenne M (1995) Immune-neuroendocrine interactions. Immunol Today 16:318–321

Tandon R, Jibson MD, Taylor SF, DeQuardo JR (1995) Conceptual models of the relationship between positive and negative symptoms. In: Shriqui L, Nasrallah HA (eds) Contemporary issues in the treatment of schizophrenia. American Psychiatric Press, Washington DC, pp 109–124

Tarazona R, González-García A, Zamzami N, Marchetti P, Frechin N, Gonzalo JA, Ruiz-Gayo M, van Rooijen N, Martínez-A. C, Kroemer G (1995) Chlorpromazine amplifies macrophage-dependent IL-10 production in vivo. J Immunol 154:861–870

van Kammen DP, Ågren H, Yao JK, O'Connor DT, Gurklis JA, Peters JL (1994) Noradrenergic activity and prediction of psychotic relapse following haloperidol withdrawal in schizophrenia. Am J Psychiatry 151:379–384

van Kammen DP, Kelley ME, Gurklis JA, Gilbertson MW, Yao JK, Peters JL (1995) Behavioral vs. biochemical prediction of clinical stability following haloperidol withdrawal in schizophrenia. Arch Gen Psychiatry 52:673–678

van Kammen DP, Kelley ME, Gurklis JA, Gilbertson MW, Yao JK, Condray R, Peters JL (1996) Predicting duration of clinical stability following haloperidol withdrawal in schizophrenia. Neuropsychopharmacology 14:275–283

Correspondence: Prof. Dr. D. P. van Kammen, Veterans Affairs Medical Center, 7180 Highland Drive, Pittsburgh, PA 15206, U.S.A.

Immunomodulatory effects of neuroleptics to the cytokine system and the cellular immune system in schizophrenia

N. Müller[1], M. Riedel[1], M. Schwarz[1], R. Gruber[2], and M. Ackenheil[1]

[1] Psychiatric Hospital and [2] Institute of Immunology, Ludwig-Maximilian University, Munich, Federal Republic of Germany

Introduction

The influence of an immune process on the pathogenesis of psychoses has been under discussion since the 1920s, when immune disturbances in schizophrenia, especially in catatonia, were reported by different authors (Bruce and Peebles, 1903; Dameshek, 1930; Lehmann-Facius, 1939).

The function of lymphocytes is determined by the pattern of the cytokines they release. Cytokines activate or recruit specific cell clones, but also mediate suppression and cell death. Cytokines also regulate signaling and communication between immune cells, the immune system, and the central nervous system (CNS), as well as within the CNS (Ransohoff and Benveniste, 1996). It has been hypothesized that activating cytokines such as Interleukin-2 (IL-2) and Interleukin-6 (IL-6) are altered in schizophrenic psychoses (Smith, 1992). The observation of schizophrenia-like symptoms, such as delusions, when cancer patients received high doses of recombinant IL-2, supports this theory (Denicoff et al., 1987).

The role of activating cytokines in the CNS

IL-2 and IL-6 are released from lymphocytes in the blood and from microglial cells or astrocytes in the CNS; they act as immunological effector cells (Plata-Salaman, 1991; Sawada et al., 1992; Ransohoff and Benveniste, 1996). Both cytokines are also actively transported into the brain (Banks and Kastin, 1992; Waguespack et al., 1994) or may cross an at least locally disturbed blood–brain barrier. Increased cytokine release in the CNS can be induced, e.g., by a viral or bacterial infection, trauma, or ischemia.

IL-2 and IL-6 in schizophrenia

Several groups of investigators have reported that the IL-2 production from lymphocytes is decreased in schizophrenic patients, and this decrease seems to be related to clinical characteristics of the patients (Ganguli et al., 1995a; Villemain et al., 1989). Decreased IL-2 production, found especially in paranoid schizophrenic patients (Wilke et al., 1996), seems to be inversely related to schizophrenic negative symptoms (Ganguli et al., 1995a). IL-2 production may also be related to an early onset of the disorder in schizophrenic patients (Ganguli et al., 1995a).

Increased IL-2 levels have also been observed in the cerebrospinal fluid (CSF) of schizophrenic patients in comparison to healthy controls (Licinio et al., 1993). Additionally, high CSF levels of IL-2 are considered a better predictor of a schizophrenic relapse than CSF levels of the catecholaminergic metabolites 5-HIAA, HVA, or psychopathological symptoms (McAllister et al., 1995). However, relapse could only be predicted on the basis of IL-2 levels in CSF, while serum levels seem not to be altered in schizophrenia.

Increased concentrations of IL-6 in the blood have been observed in patients suffering from schizophrenia (Ganguli et al., 1994; Maes et al., 1994). Higher sIL-6R levels are related to paranoid-hallucinatory symptoms (Müller et al., 1997a). In contrast to sIL-2R, sIL-6R do not bind and inactivate IL-6, but rather form a complex with IL-6 which enhances the biological activity of the latter via a signal-transducing protein (Mackiewicz et al., 1992). The same process also occurs in the CNS (Schöbitz et al., 1995).

Cytokines and catecholaminergic neurotransmission

The significance of IL-2 and IL-6 in schizophrenia can be explained by their influence on catecholaminergic neurotransmission. Data from basic research suggest that IL-6 strongly influences the dopaminergic system. In-vitro studies have shown that the stimulation of neuronal cells by IL-6 leads to increased release of dopamine (Hama et al., 1991). Animal studies revealed that the application of IL-6 in the peripheral blood leads to increased dopamine turnover in the frontal cortex and hippocampus (Zalcman et al., 1994). The hippocampus – one of the CNS structures involved in schizophrenia – has the most pronounced expression of IL-6 receptors. Accordingly, there are parallel findings for IL-2. The pyramidal layer of the hippocampus shows also an high density for IL-2 receptors (Plata-Salaman and Ffrench-Mullen, 1993). Peripheral application of IL-2 causes an increase of catecholaminergic neurotransmission in the hippocampus and frontal cortex (Zalcman et al., 1994).

Neuroleptics – immune effects to soluble cytokine receptors

If an increased concentration of activating cytokines in the CNS is involved in schizophrenia, a suppressive effect of antipsychotic treatment on these cytokines would be expected. Earlier studies have reported immunosuppressive effects of neuroleptics (Saunders and Muchmore, 1964; Baker et al., 1977; Maes et al., 1994). However, the term immunosuppression is a vague and general; the effects need to be specified. Other studies, in contrast, have not detected any suppression of the immune system (Müller et al., 1991). Some in vitro investigations have even observed an immune activating function of neuroleptics (Gallien et al., 1977; Zarrabi et al., 1979). These contradictory results indicate, that in vitro and in vivo effects, as well as short-term and long-term effects must be differentiated (McAllister et al., 1989; Rapaport et al., 1990). Moreover, since the immune system is composed of complex regulatory mechanisms, the effects of its different components must be specified.

Since increased sIL-2R levels have been reported in schizophrenics (Ganguli and Rabin, 1989; Maes et al., 1996; Rapaport et al., 1989, 1993, 1994), we investigated the role of neuroleptic medication. Three studies dealt with patients treated with neuroleptics at the time of inclusion in the study (Ganguli and Rabin, 1989; Rapaport et al., 1989, 1993); thus, a treatment effect cannot be excluded. Only one study of schizophrenic patients without neuroleptic treatment showed increased levels of sIL-2R (Rapaport et al., 1994). Since these patients were Koreans, not Caucasians, racial or other genetic factors may have played a role. Indeed, Korean patients showed significantly different sIL-2R serum levels than Caucasians (Rapaport et al., 1994).

Increased sIL-2R levels in the group of neuroleptic-treated schizophrenic patients compared with those in controls, however, were also observed in our study, probably being due to a treatment effect (Müller et al., 1997b). An increase of sIL-2R during neuroleptic treatment was described before, especially for clozapine (Pollmächer et al., 1995), and risperidone (Maes et al., 1996). In our patient group, this increase was not restricted to clozapine or risperidone but also occurred in patients receiving other neuroleptics. This agrees with the finding that sIL-2R levels did not differ in neuroleptic-treated patients regardless of whether they received clozapine, haloperidole, or fluphenazine (Ganguli et al., 1995b). The fact that the acute single dose administration of 5 or 10 mg haloperidol influences not sIL-2R levels (Rapaport et al., 1991) interferes not with the observation of an increase of sIL-2R during long term therapy with neuroleptics including haloperidol under naturalistic clinical conditions.

The decrease of sIL-6R levels during neuroleptic treatment and decreased sIL-6R levels in neuroleptic-medicated schizophrenics compared with controls in parallel to increased sIL-2R (Müller et al., 1997b) also implies a down-regulation of an immune-activating compound. As discussed above, sIL-6R enhances the biological activity of IL-6. Whereas neuroleptic treatment has a down-regulating effect on sIL-6R levels in schizophrenic patients (Maes et al., 1995), it has also had an inhibiting effect on the m-RNA of activating cytokines (Schleuning et al., 1989) as well as the release of cytokines in vitro (Schleuning et al., 1994). Inhibitory effects of chlorpromazine, slightly also of other neuroleptics (haloperidol, fluphenazine), on the TNF production were also observed in animal experiments (Bertini et al., 1993). Moreover, chlorpromazine protects from IL-1-toxicity and endotoxin induced TNF-toxicity in mice, too (Bertini et al., 1989).

Effects of neuroleptics to the CNS cytokine-network

Our results indicate that neuroleptics act immunosuppressively by inhibiting of IL-2 and IL-6 via their soluble receptors (Müller et al., 1997b). There are three possible explanations for these effects. First, the most simple and intriguing possibility is that the same effect takes place in the CNS. Second, it is possible that less IL-2 is transported across the BBB, because a larger amount is bound to molecules that cannot easily cross the BBB. In parallel, less IL-6 is activated by the complex IL-6/sIL-6R. Third, since neuroleptic treatment seems to increase the permeability of the BBB for certain compounds (Müller et al., 1997b) more sIL-2R may cross the BBB and inhibit further activation by IL-2. SIL-6R, however, may be less available despite increased BBB permeability. These suggested functional peripheral immune system-CNS interactions in schizophrenia are still speculative, but much evidence including the interactions of IL-2, IL-6, and the catecholaminergic neurotransmission, supports this view.

Possible impaired antigen presentation and recognition in schizophrenia

The question arises as to sIL-2R and sIL-6R serum levels do not differ between untreated schizophrenics and controls (Maes et al., 1994, 1996; Müller et al., 1997b). A disturbance of the cytokine network within the CNS may not necessarily be accompanied by a disturbed cytokine system within the peripheral immune system, especially when the blood–brain barrier is intact. It has been suggested that untreated schizophrenics may have a defect in the presentation or recognition of antigens by T lymphocytes (Müller et al., 1991, 1997c; Russo et al., 1994), hypothetically associated with a relative lack of activation of the peripheral immune system, a lack in peripheral immune system-CNS communication, and an insufficient control of activating cytokines in the CNS by the peripheral immune system.

The increase of sIL-2R receptors, however, indicates that neuroleptics have immunomodulatory effects. Increased serum concentrations of sIL-2R lead to increased concentrations of sIL-2R in the CSF, since the diffusion of proteins across the blood–brain barrier depends on serum concentrations (Reiber and Felgenhauer, 1987). In case of a disturbance of the blood-brain barrier (the case in about 1/3 of the schizophrenic patients), sIL-2R can pass through it. Increased sIL-2R could mediate an immunosuppressive effect due to its capacity to bind IL-2 and thus reduce its availability (Barral-Netto et al., 1991; Brivio et al., 1991). Increase in sIL-2R, however, is also an (unspecific) effect of immunosuppressive drugs, such as cyclosporin A (Hornung et al., 1992).

Treatment with neuroleptics is associated with differentiated regulatory effects on the cytokines in the peripheral immune system. In view of interactions between the cytokines in the peripheral immune system and in the CNS, on the one hand, and of the cytokines and the catecholaminergic neurotransmission in CNS regions critical for schizophrenia, on the other, it seems necessary to consider the immunoregulatory effects of neuroleptics when determining the therapeutic efficacy of treatment for schizophrenia (Müller and Ackenheil, 1997).

Improvement of antigen-presentation/recognition by neuroleptic therapy?

In a recent study, we estimated the expression of the adhesion molecule receptors very late antigen-4 (VLA-4) and leucocyte function antigen-1 (LFA-1) on T-helper- (CD4$^+$) and on T-suppressor/cytotoxic-(CD8$^+$) lymphocytes in schizophrenic patients before and during neuroleptic treatment compared to controls (Müller et al., 1997b). Adhesion is mediated by a multiple receptor-ligand system. The very late antigen-4 (VLA-4) belongs to the β1, and the lymphocyte function-related antigen-1 (LFA-1) to the β2 integrins. Adhesion molecules are expressed on endothelial cells, and the expression on endothelial cells is increased by activating cytokines (DeVries et al., 1994). Adhesion molecules are also expressed on parenchymal cells, in the CNS, e.g. VCAM-1 (Vascular Adhesion Molecule), the ligand of VLA-4, and ICAM-1 (Intra Cellular Adhesion Molecule), the ligand of LFA-1, on astrocytes and microglial cells, but also on neurons (Fabry et al., 1994; Héry et al., 1995; Hampel et al., 1996). This system has three functions: (1) accumulation of lymphocytes in the vessels of the target organ by adhesion, (2) diapedesis through the endothelium of certain lymphocyte subpopulations, and (3) traffic into the parenchyma (Raine et al., 1990; Oppenheimer-Marks et al., 1991; DeVries et al., 1994).

However, during neuroleptic treatment and psychopathological improvement there was a significant increase in the expression of VLA-4 on CD4$^+$ cells and on CD8$^+$ cells, while in unmedicated patients there was no difference to controls regarding the percentage of CD4$^+$- and CD8$^+$-lymphocytes and the expression of adhesion molecules on lymphocytes. Moreover, another study of the cellular immune system revealed increased cytotoxic T-memory cells (CD8$^+$CD45RO$^+$) in nonmedicated schizophrenics before neuroleptic treatment and an increase of CD4$^+$CD45RO$^+$ and CD4$^+$HLADR$^+$ lymphocytes during treatment with neuroleptics (Gruber et al., 1997). This finding indicates that activated CD4$^+$-lymphocytes increase during neuroleptic therapy. Furthermore, it suggests a functional influence of CD45RO$^+$ T-suppressor/cytotoxic cells in schizophrenia and a regulatory influence of neuroleptic treatment on the helper function of CD45RO$^+$ T-cells. Certain subsets of CD8$^+$CD45RO$^+$-cells seem to exhibit high transendothelial migratory capacity (Berman et al., 1995), a feature that would be expected in cells crossing the blood–brain barrier. Moreover, the number of the CD8$^+$-CD45RO$^+$-cells is related to schizophrenic "positive symptoms" (such as delusions, hallucinations, formal thought disorder, and disorganized behavior) which do not improve in patients with high CD8$^+$CD45RO$^+$-cells under therapy (Gruber et al., 1997). Especially the patients which only show a poor response to neuroleptic therapy show high CD8$^+$CD45RO$^+$-cells. The increase of CD4$^+$HLADR$^+$ and the CD4$^+$CD45RO$^+$-cells also seems to reflect a therapeutic effect. Since a defect in the recognition or presentation of antigens may play a role in schizophrenia (Müller et al., 1991; Russo et al., 1995), an improvement in antigen presentation or recognition may be an immunological mechanism that is involved in clinical improvement during antipsychotic treatment. Experimental data show that antigen presentation and recognition can be impaired by viral mechanisms (De Val et al., 1989; Townsend et al., 1988; Niewiesk et al., 1993). Possibly, treatment with neuroleptics improves the presentation and/or recognition of antigens. The increase of the CD4$^+$HLADR$^+$ and the CD4$^+$CD45RO$^+$-cells may reflect this improvement, especially, since CD4$^+$ cells mediate the specific answer to an antigen presented by antigen presenting cells.

A speculative model of immunomodulatory effects of neuroleptics

While the upregulation of CD4$^+$ lymphocytes (CD4$^+$HLADR$^+$, CD4$^+$-CD45RO$^+$, VLA-4$^+$/CD4$^+$) provides help, presents antigens via the HLA-class II complex, and secretes activating cytokines, CD8$^+$ lymphocytes can influence other immune competent cells and their cytokine production in two different ways:

1. It has been shown that HLA-class I dependent specific cytotoxic T-

lymphocytes (CD8$^+$-cells) can enter organs and regulate the gene expression of parenchymal cells (dependent on cytokines and delayed in onset) without destroying these cells (Guidotti et al., 1994) or

2. They can act cytotoxically, leading to the destruction of certain cell types.

One can speculate that certain invading clones of cytotoxic lymphocytes influence the production of activating cytokines in the CNS (Licinio et al., 1993; McAllister et al., 1995) by binding to activated astrocytes or microglia cells in the CNS. In this context it must be recalled that the ligand of the VLA-4$^+$ cells, VCAM-1, shows a higher expression on neurons than on astrocytes in vitro (Hery et al., 1995).

In parallel, neuroleptic treatment exhibits direct influence to activating cytokines, possibly not only in the peripheral immune system, but primarily to the cytokine-network in the CNS. While the improvement of antigen-presentation and -recognition may lead to an upregulation of the specific HLA-class II mediated immune answer and to a functional downregulation of cytotoxic T-cells, this activation of the T-helper cell system may lead to an overactivation of the immune system in certain cases and induce an autoimmune process in a subgroup of schizophrenics. An autoimmune process is postulated in about one third of schizophrenic patients (Ganguli et al., 1987; Müller and Ackenheil, 1995a). Such an autoimmune process might be supported by an increased permeability of the blood–brain barrier, because further activating components of the immune system may cross the blood–brain barrier, too.

Acknowledgements

This work was supported by a grant of the Volkswagen Foundation to M. A. and N. M. (I 69/356–357).

References

Baker GA, Syntalo R, Blumenstein J (1977) Effects of psychotropic agents upon the blastogenic response on human T-lymphocytes. Biol Psychiatry 12:159–169

Banks WA, Kastin AJ (1992) The interleukins-1 alpha, -1 beta, and -2 do not acutely disrupt the murine blood-brain barrier. Int J Immunopharmacol 14:629–636

Barral-Netto M, Barral A, Santos SB, Carvalho EM, Badaro R, Rocha H, Reed SG, Johnson WD jr (1991) Soluble IL-2 receptors as an agent of serum-mediated suppression in human visceral leishmaniasis. J Immunol 147:281–284

Berman JS, Mahoney K, Saukkonen JJ, Masuyama J (1995) Migration of distinct subsets of CD8+ blood cells through endothelial cell monolayers in vitro. J Leukoc Biol 58:317–324

Bertini S, Bianchi M, Mengozzi M, Ghezzi P (1989) Protective effect of chlorpromazine against the lethality of interleukin 1 in adrenalectomized or actinomycin D-sensitized mice. Biochem Biophys Res Commun 165:942–947

Bertini S, Garattini R, Delgado P, Ghezzi P (1993) Pharmacological activities of chlorpromazine involved in the inhibition of tumour necrosis factor production in vivo in mice. Immunology 79:217–219

Brivio S, Lissoni P, Mancini D, Tisi E, Tancini G, Barni S, Nociti V (1991) Effect of antitumor surgery on soluble interleukin-2 receptor serum levels. Am J Surg 161: 466–469

Bruce LC, Peebles AMS (1903) Clinical and experimental observations on catatonia. J Ment Sci 49:614–628

Burkly LC, Jakubowski A, Newman BM, Rosa MD, Chi-Rosso G, Lobb RR (1991) Signaling by vascular cell adhesion molecule-1 (VCAM-1) through VLA-4 promotes CD3-dependent T cell proliferation. Eur J Immunol 21:2871–2875

Dameshek W (1930) White blood cells in dementia praecox and dementia paralytica. Arch Neurol Psychiatry 24:855

Denicoff KD, Rubinoff DR, Papa MZ, Simpson C, Seipp CA, Lotze MT, Chang AE, Rosenstein D, Rosenberg SA (1987) The neuropsychiatric effects of treatment with interleukin-2 and lymphokine-activated killer cells. Ann Intern Med 107: 293–300

Del Val M, Münch K, Reddehase MJ, Koszinowski UH (1991) Presentation of CMV immediate-early antigen to cytolytic T lymphocytes is selectively prevented by viral genes expressed in the early phase. Cell 58:305–315

De Vries HE, Moor ACE, Blom-Roosemalen MCM, de Broer AG, Breimer DD, van Berkel TJC, Kuiper J (1994) Lymphocyte adhesion to brain capillary endothelial cells in vitro. J Neuroimmunol 52:1–8

Fabry Z, Raine CS, Hart MN (1994) Nervous tissue as an immune compartment: the dialect of the immune response in the CNS. Immunol Today 15:218–224

Gallien M, Schnetzler JP, Morin J (1977) Antinuclear antibodies and lupus cells in 600 hospitalized phenothiazine treated patients. Ann Med Psychol Med 1:237–248

Ganguli R, Rabin BS (1989) Increased serum interleukin 2 receptor levels in schizophrenic and brain damaged subjects. Arch Gen Psychiatry 46:292

Ganguli R, Rabin BS, Kelly RH, Lyte M, Ragu U (1987) Clinical and laboratory evidence of autoimmunity in acute schizophrenia. Ann NY Acad Sci 496:676–685

Ganguli R, Yang Z, Shurin G, Chengappa R, Brar JS, Gubbi AV, Rabin BS (1994) Serum interleukin-6 concentration in schizophrenia: elevation associated with duration of illness. Psychiatry Res 51:1–10

Ganguli R, Brar JS, Chengappa KR, DeLeo M, Yang ZW, Shurin G, Rabin B (1995a) Mitogen-stimulated interleukin 2 production in never-medicated, first episode schizophrenics – the influence of age of onset and negative symptoms. Arch Gen Psychiatry 52:878

Ganguli R, Brar JS, Rabin BS (1995b) Reply on: Pollmächer T et al.: Clozapine-induced increase in plasma levels of soluble interleukin-2 receptors. Arch Gen Psychiatry 52:668–672

Gruber R, Hadjamu M, Riedel M, Schwarz M, Primbs J, Ackenheil M, Müller N

(1997c) CD8⁺ memory T-lymphocytes (CD45RO⁺) are elevated in unmedicated schizophrenic patients while CD4⁺CD45RO⁺ and CD4⁺HLADR⁺ T-cells increase during treatment with neuroleptics. Am J Psychiatry (submitted)

Guidotti LC, Ando K, Hobbs MV, Ishikawa T, Runkel L, Schreiber RD, Chisari FV (1994) Cytotoxic T lymphocytes inhibit hepatitis B virus gene expression by a noncytolytic mechanism in transgenic mice. Proc Natl Acad Sci USA 91:3764–3768

Hama T, Kushima Y, Miyamoto M, Kubota M, Takei N, Hatanaka H (1991) Interleukin-6 improves the survival of mesencephalic catecholaminergic and septal cholinergic neurons from post-natal, two-week-old rats in cultures. Neurosci 40: 445–452

Hampel H, Schwarz M, Kötter HU, Schneider C, Müller N (1996) Cell adhesion molecules in the central nervous system. Drug News & Perspect 9:69–81

Héry C, Sébire G, Peudenier S, Tardieu M (1995) Adhesion to human neurons and astrocytes of monocytes: the role of interaction of CR3 and ICAM-1 and modulating by cytokines. J Neuroimmunol 57:101–109

Hornberg M, Arolt V, Wilke I, Kruse A, Kirchner H (1995) Production of interferons and lymphokines in leukocyte cultures of patients with schizophrenia. Schizophr Res 15:237–242

Hornung N, Raskova J, Raska K, Degiannis D (1992) Il-2 responsiveness of lectin-induced lymphoblasts: soluble IL-2 receptor release and differential in vitro effects of immunosuppressants. Int J Immunopharmacol 14:753–760

Licinio J, Seibyl JP, Altemus M, Charney DS, Krystal JH (1993) Elevated levels of interleukin-2 in neuroleptic-free schizophrenics. Am J Psychiatry 150:1408–1410

Lehmann-Facius H (1939) Serologisch-analytische Versuche mit Liquores und Seren von Schizophrenen. Allg Z Psychiatrie 110:232–243

Mackiewicz A, Schooltink H, Heinrich PC, Rose-John S (1992) Complex of soluble human IL-6-receptor/IL-6 up-regulates expression of acute-phase proteins. J Immunol 49:2021–2027

Maes M, Meltzer HY, Bosmans E (1994) Immune-inflammatory markers in schizophrenia: comparison to normal controls and effects of clozapine. Acta Psychiatr Scand 89:346–351

Maes M, Bosmans E, Ranjan R, Vandoolaeghe B, Meltzer HY, De Ley M, Berghmans R, Stans G, Desnyder R (1996) Lower plasma CC16, a natural anti-inflammatory protein, and increased plasma interleukin-1 receptor antagonist in schizophrenia: effects of antipsychotic drugs. Schizophr Res 21:39–50

McAllister CG, Rapaport MH, Pickar D, Paul SM (1989) Effect of short term administration of antipsychotic drugs on lymphocyte subsets in schizophrenic patients. Arch Gen Psychiatry 46:956–957

McAllister CG, van Kammen DP, Rehn TJ, Miller AN, Gurklis J, Kelley ME, Yao J, Peters JL (1995) Increases in CSF levels of interleukin-2 in schizophrenia: effects of recurrance of psychosis and medication status. Am J Psychiatry 152:1291–1297

Müller N, Ackenheil M (1995a) The immune system and schizophrenia. In: Leonard BE, Miller K (eds) Stress, the immune system and psychiatry. Wiley and Sons, Chichester, pp 137–164

Müller N, Ackenheil M (1995b) Immunoglobulin and albumin contents of cerebrospinal fluid in schizophrenic patients: the relationship to negative symptomatology. Schizophr Res 14:223–228

Müller N, Ackenheil M (1997) Psychoneuroimmunology and the cytokine action in the CNS: implications for psychiatric disorders. Prog Neuropsychopharmacol Biol Psychiatry (in press)

Müller N, Ackenheil M, Hofschuster E, Mempel W, Eckstein R (1991) Cellular immunity in schizophrenic patients before and during neuroleptic therapy. Psychiatry Res 37:147–160

Müller N, Dobmeier P, Empl M, Riedel M, Schwarz M, Ackenheil M (1997) Soluble IL-6 receptors in the serum and cerebrospinal fluid of paranoid schizophrenic patients. Eur Psychiatry 12:294–299

Müller N, Empl M, Riedel M, Schwarz M, Ackenheil M (1997b) Decrease of soluble IL-6 receptor- and increase of soluble IL-2 receptor serum levels in schizophrenic patients reflect the immunomodulatory effect of neuroleptics. Eur Arch Psychiatry Clin Neurosci (in press)

Müller N, Hadjamu M, Riedel M, Primbs J, Ackenheil M, Gruber R (1997c) Adhesion-molecule receptor expression on T-cells and the role of the blood–brain barrier in schizophrenia. Am J Psychiatry (submitted)

Niewiesk S, Brinckmann U, Bankamp B, Sirak S, Liebert UG, ter Meulen V (1993) Susceptibility to measles virus-induced encephalitis in mice correlates with impaired antigen presentation to cytotoxic T-lymphocytes. J Virol 67:75–81

Oppenheimer-Marks N, Davis LS, Bogue DT, Ramberg J, Lipsky PE (1991) Differential utilisation of ICAM-1 and VCAM-1 during the adhesion and transendothelial migration of human T-lymphocytes. J Immunol 147:2913–2921

Plata-Salaman CR, Ffrench-Mullen JM (1993) Interleukin-2 modulates calcium currents in dissociated hippocampal CA1 neurons. Neuroreport 4:579–581

Pollmächer T, Hinze-Selch D, Mullington J, Holsboer F (1995) Clozapine-induced increase in plasma levels of soluble interleukin-2 receptors. Arch Gen Psychiatry 52:877–878

Raine CS, Canella B, Duijvestijn AM, Cross AH (1990) Homing to central nervous vasculature by antigen-specific lymphocytes. II Lymphocyte/endothelial cell adhesion during the initial stages of autoimmune demyelination. Lab Invest 63:476–479

Ransohoff RM, Benveniste EN (1996) Cytokines and the CNS. CNC Press NY, London

Rapaport MH, McAllister CG, Pickar D, Nelson DM, Paul SM (1989) Elevated levels of soluble interleukin 2 receptors in schizophrenia. Arch Gen Psychiatry 46:292

Rapaport MH, McAllister CG, Kirch DG, Pickar D (1990) The effects of typical and atypical neuroleptics on mitogen-induced T lymphocyte responsiveness. Biol Psychiatry 29:715–717

Rapaport MH, Torrey EF, McAllister CG, Nelson DM, Pickar D, Paul SM (1993) Increased serum soluble interleukin-2 receptors in schizophrenic monozygotic twins. Eur Arch Psychiatry Clin Neurosci 243:7–10

Rapaport MH, McAllister CG, Kim YS, Han JH, Pickar D, Nelson DM, Kirch DG, Paul SM (1994) Increased soluble interleukin-2 receptors in caucasian and korean schizophrenic patients. Biol Psychiatry 35:767–771

Reiber H, Felgenhauer K (1987) Protein transfer at the blood cerebrospinal fluid barrier and the quantitation of the humoral immune response within the central nervous system. Clin Chem Acta 163:319–328

Russo R, Ciminale M, Ditommaso S, Siliquini R, Zotti C, Ruggenini AM (1994) Hepatitis B vaccination in psychiatric patients. Lancet 343:394

Saunders JC, Muchmore E (1964) Phenothiazine effect on human antibody synthesis. Br J Psychiatry 110:84–89

Sawada M, Suzumura A, Marunouchi T (1992) TNF-alpha induces IL-6 production by astrocytes, but not by microglia. Brain Res 583:296–299

Schleuning MJ, Duggan A, Reem GH (1989) Inhibition by chlorpromazine of lymphokine-specific m-RNA expression in human thymocytes. Eur J Immunol 19: 1491–1496

Schleuning M, Brumme V, Wilmanns W (1994) Inhibition of cyclosporin A/FK 506 resistant, lymphokine-induced T-cell activation by phenothiazine derivates. Naunyn Schmiedebergs Arch Pharmacol 350:100–103

Schöbitz B, Pezeshki G, Pohl T, Hermann U, Heinrich PC, Holsboer F, Reul JM (1995) Soluble interleukin-6 (IL-6) receptor augments central effects of IL-6 in vivo. FASEB J 9:659–664

Smith RS (1992) A comprehensive macrophage-T-lymphocyte theory of schizophrenia. Med Hypotheses 39:248–257

Townsend A, Bastin J, Gold K, Brownlee G, Andrew B, Coupar B, Boyle D, Chan S, Smith G (1988) Defective presentation to class I-restricted cytotoxic T lymphocytes in vaccinia-infected cells is overcome by enhanced degradation of antigen. J Exp Med 168:1211–1224

Villemain F, Chatenoud L, Galinowski A, Homo-Delarche F, Genestet D, Loo H, Zarifarain E, Bach JF (1989) Aberrant T-cell-mediated immunity in untreated schizophrenic patients: deficient interleukin-2 production. Am J Psychiatry 146: 609–616

Waguespack PJ, Banks WA, Kastin AJ (1994) Interleukin-2 does not cross the blood–brain-barrier by a saturable transport system. Brain Res Bull 34:103–109

Wilke I, Arolt V, Rothermundt M, Weitzsch C, Hornberg M, Kirchner H (1996) Investigations of cytokine production in whole blood cultures of paranoid and residual schizophrenic patients. Eur Arch Psychiatry Clin Neurosci 246:279–284

Zarrabi MH, Zucker S, Miller F, Derman RM, Romeno GS, Hartnett JA, Varma AO (1979) Immunologic and coagulation disorders in chlorpromazine-treated patients. Ann Intern Med 91:194–199

Zalcman S, Green-Johnson JM, Murray L, Nance DM, Dyck D, Anisman H, Greenberg AH (1994) Cytokine-specific central monoamine alterations induced by interleukin-1, -2 and -6. Brain Res 643:40–49

Correspondence: Priv.-Doz. Dr. med. Dipl. Psych. N. Müller, Psychiatric Hospital, University of Munich, Nußbaumstrasse 7, D-80336 München, Federal Republic of Germany.

Cytokines in schizophrenia.
Results from a longitudinal study

M. Rothermundt[1], V. Arolt[1], C. Weitzsch[1], D. Eckhoff[2], and H. Kirchner[2]

Departments of [1] Psychiatry and [2] Immunology and Transfusion Medicine, University of Lübeck School of Medicine, Lübeck, Federal Republic of Germany

Introduction

Several lines of evidence indicate that an immunological dysfunction may contribute to the multifactoral etiology of schizophrenia (Kirch, 1993; Syvälahti, 1994; Wright et al., 1993). One approach to further investigate this dysfunction focuses on the field of cytokines. Cytokines are protein mediators that are produced by leukocytes. There is a complex interaction between the different immunocompetent cells, their products and mediators. Cytokines regulate the differentiation and activation of the immunologically active cells and can be regarded as functional markers of cellular immunity.

Research efforts concerning cytokines in schizophrenia have yielded increasingly consistent results. In 1983 Kolyaskina showed a reduced proliferative activity of T-lymphocytes after mitogen induction. It has been reported by several groups (including our own) that the production of interleukin-2 (IL-2) by lymphocytes after stimulation is significantly lower in schizophrenics than in non-psychotic controls (Bessler et al., 1995; Ganguli et al., 1989, 1992, 1995; Hornberg et al., 1995; Rothermundt et al., 1996; Villemain et al., 1989). The decreased IL-2 production in acutely ill schizophrenics compared to remitted ones suggests that IL-2 is a state marker of acute illness rather than a trait marker (Ganguli et al., 1993). Serum levels of IL-2 have been found to be unchanged (Barak et al., 1995; Gattaz et al., 1992). In the cerebrospinal fluid (CSF) of schizophrenics IL-2 was found to be unchanged (El-Mallakh et al., 1993; Barak et al., 1995) or elevated (Licinio et al., 1993). McAllister et al. (1995) showed higher IL-2 levels in the CSF of schizophrenic patients who relapsed than in those who remained in a remitted state.

Despite the close functional relationship between IL-2 and Interferon gamma (IFN-γ) (the production of IFN-γ is stimulated by IL-2) the results concerning IFN-γ in schizophrenia so far are less impressive than those regarding IL-2. A tendency towards a decreased production after stimulation has been reported (Hornberg et al., 1995; Katila et al., 1989;

Moises et al., 1985). Serum levels of IFN-γ do not seem to be elevated (Becker et al., 1990; Gattaz et al., 1992; Schindler et al., 1986) with the exception of higher levels reported by Preble and Torrey (1985). It is noteworthy, however, that in these studies a range of schizophrenic subtypes were included, and acute as well as remitted schizophrenics have often been compiled in the same samples. Wilke et al. (1996) showed a decreased IFN-γ production in acutely ill schizophrenics compared to healthy controls while remitted schizophrenics showed no difference in IFN-γ production after stimulation.

It has been hypothesized that a decreased in vitro stimulated IL-2 production is most probably a manifestation of exhaustion of the TH1 subset of CD4 positive cells' capacity to synthesize IL-2 consequent on in vivo overproduction (Ganguli et al., 1993; Kroemer and Wick, 1989). However, another possibility has to be considered. IFN-γ and IL-2 are produced by TH-1 lymphocytes. TH-2 lymphocytes and their products (e.g. Interleukin 10 (IL-10)) are regarded as antagonists of the TH-1 system. Therefore one could imagine that the decreased production of IL-2 and IFN-γ after stimulation is due to an upregulation of TH-2 cytokines (Mosmann and Moore, 1991; Romagnani, 1991, 1992; Scott and Kaufmann, 1991; Zlotnik and Moore, 1991).

Another important question is to what extent the decreased production of IL-2 and IFN-γ after stimulation could be explained by differing cortisol levels in those patients. Ganguli et al. (1993) showed that serum cortisol was significantly higher in patients with low IL-2 production. A negative correlation between cortisol and IL-2 production was demonstrated only in autoantibody positive patients. Sasaki et al. (1994) observed normal cortisol levels on admission but increased levels after 8 weeks of treatment.

Considering the differing results of acutely ill and remitted schizophrenic patients it seems to be of value to imply a longitudinal study that monitors acutely ill patients on their way to clinical improvement and remission.

In order to clarify the earlier findings and to expand the knowledge on the cytokine production in schizophrenia and further elucidate the immunological dysfunction we conducted a study on a homogenous group of acutely ill schizophrenic inpatients. These patients were psychiatrically and immunologically investigated on hospital admission and followed up closely. TH1 as well as TH2 cytokines and cortisol levels were measured.

Materials and methods

Patients and controls

Blood samples were taken from 44 patients (23 men, 21 women) hospitalized in the Department of Psychiatry, School of Medicine, University of Lübeck suffering from an acute exacerbation of schizophrenia. They were clinically diagnosed by two psychiatrists according to DSM-III-R and ICD-10 criteria. The mean age of the patients and controls was 34.7 respectively 34.8 years with a range between 17 and 62 years. The mean age of disease onset was 26.2 years. 22 patients were up to 30 years of age and 22 were older than 30. Acute infectious diseases were excluded by measuring the body temperature, C-reactive protein and erythrocyte sedimentation rate. All but 4 patients received neuroleptic medication prior to admission. The control group consisted of 44 healthy blood donors. Patients and controls were matched as pairs concerning age, sex, and race and investigated concomitantly on the same day. The first investigation took place on the day after admission to the hospital (T1). 2 (T2) and 4 weeks (T3) thereafter they were reinvestigated.

Whole-blood assay

Heparinized blood was drawn by vein puncture from patients and controls, stored at 4 °C and cultured in a whole-blood assay within 1–2 hours according to a technique previously described (Kirchner et al., 1982). In a 5 ml polysterole tube (Greiner, Nürtingen, Germany) 100 μl of blood was added to 850 μl of Roswell Park Memorial Institute (RPMI) medium (Biochrom, Berlin, Germany) supplemented with 2 mmol L-glutamine, 100 U/ml of penicillin, and 100 μl/ml of streptomycin (Gibco, Karlsruhe, Germany). For the induction of IL-2, IL-10, and IFN-γ, phytohemagglutinin (PHA) (Borroughs Wellcome, Dartford, Great Britain) was added at a concentration of 1.78 mitogenic units (0.1 mg/ml). The blood suspension was incubated at 37 °C/5% CO_2 for 48 h (IL-2), 72 h (IL-10), or 96 h (IFN-γ), respectively. The supernatants were recovered and kept frozen at -80 °C.

Determination of cytokines and cortisol

Cytokine concentrations in the supernatants and cortisol levels in the serum were determined by enzyme-linked immunosorbent assay (ELISA) technique. Recombinant cytokines were used as standards. We used ELISA kits from BioSource International, Camarillo, USA, carried out according to the manufacturer's instructions. The intraassay coefficients were 4.5% for IFN-γ, 5.7% for IL-10 and 5.8% for IL-2. The interassay coefficients were 5.7% for IFN-γ, 5.4% for IL-10 and 7.2% for IL-2.

Table 1

	T1	T2	T3	controls	p
Interferon gamma in pg/ml	2254.0 ±2897.6	3628.4 ±4782.0	3501.4 ±2551.9	5611.7 ±5315.3	≤ 0.001
Interleukin 2 in pg/ml	127.6 ±120.6	182.3 ±170.3	144.2 ±126.3	257.8 ±237.6	≤ 0.005
Interleukin 10 in pg/ml	166.5 ±117.4			285.9 ±261.9	n. s.
Cortisol in nmol/l	444.7 ±148.5	400.7 ±102.2	390.2 ±113.4	374.5 ±122.8	n. s.

Statistics

The Wilcoxon Matched-Pairs Signed-Ranks Test and the Friedman Two-Way Anova Test provided by the SPSS-PC program were used for statistical evaluation.

Results

The production of IFN-γ by schizophrenics (Table 1, Fig. 1) was significantly decreased at all three points of investigation during the 4 weeks of the study with a minimum on admission ($p \leq 0.001$). After dividing the group according to age the level of significance for all points of investigation was only reached for patients older than 30 years of age ($p \leq 0.01$). The younger schizophrenics had significantly ($p < 0.05$)

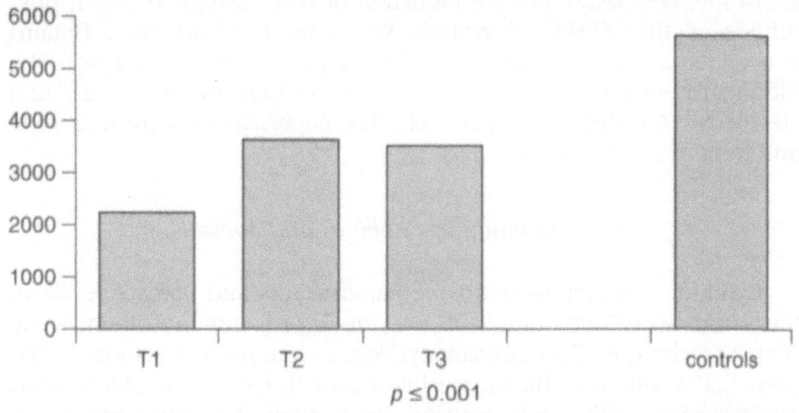

$p \leq 0.001$

Fig. 1. Interferon gamma in pg/ml

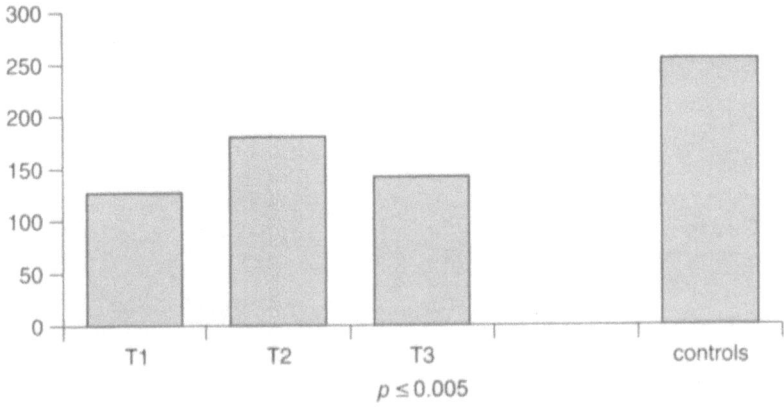

Fig. 2. Interleukin 2 in pg/ml

lower IFN-γ production on admission and a tendency towards a decreased production after 2 and 4 weeks ($p \leq 0.01$). Female patients as well as controls showed a lower production than males ($p \leq 0.01$).

The IL-2 production (Table 1, Fig. 2) was also significantly lowered at all points of investigation ($p \leq 0.005$). Younger patients (≤ 30 years of age) as well as older ones (> 30 years of age) showed decreased levels at all points of investigation ($p \leq 0.05$ and $p \leq 0.05$ respectively). No sex difference was detected. There was a correlation among the schizophrenic patients between the IL-2 production at all points of investigation ($p \leq 0.05$). Both, IFN-γ and IL-2 production maximally impaired on admission followed by an increase after 2 and 4 weeks of inpatient treatment.

The production of IL-10 (Table 1, Fig. 3) after mitogen stimulation showed no significant difference between the patients and controls. Results of T2 and T3 were not available. These results did not depend on age or sex.

All patients showed normal serum cortisol levels at all three points of investigation (Table 1). There was no difference between patients and controls as well as no differences concerning age and sex were detected. No correlation between cortisol levels and cytokine production at any point of investigation was found.

Discussion

The results of this study support the hypothesis that schizophrenia might be associated with an immunological dysfunction. Concerning interleukin-2, the results of our study confirm the previously described

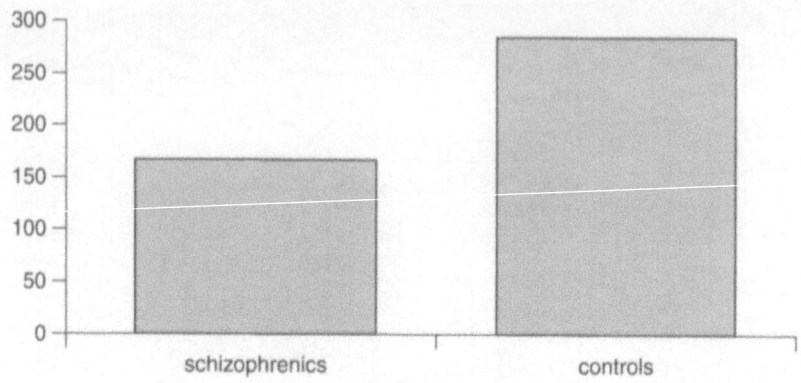

Fig. 3. Interleukin 10 in pg/ml

impaired ability of the T-cells to produce IL-2 after mitogen stimulation in acutely ill schizophrenic patients (Bessler et al., 1995; Ganguli et al., 1989, 1992, 1995; Hornberg et al., 1995; Rothermundt et al., 1996; Villemain et al., 1989). IFN-γ seems to be an equally stable parameter regarding the immunological dysfunction in schizophrenics.

There is a slight increase of the IL-2 and IFN-γ production after 2 weeks of inpatient treatment followed by a decrease after 4 weeks, but these differences are not statistically significant. Since the point of time of the hospital admission does not give information concerning the onset of an acute schizophrenic episode and the investigation period of 4 weeks is too short we cannot further comment on the hypothesis that IL-2 is a state rather than a trait marker of the illness (Ganguli et al., 1993), but in two previously published studies our group confirmed this hypothesis for IFN-γ (Rothermundt et al., 1996; Wilke et al., 1996). The lower production of IFN-γ by females compared to males previously described by Kita et al. (1991) is confirmed by our study for healthy and schizophrenic women.

According to the hypothesis of antagonism between TH-1 and TH-2 cytokines (Mosmann and Moore, 1991; Romagnani, 1991, 1992; Scott and Kaufmann, 1991; Zlotnik and Moore, 1991) one would expect an upregulation of TH-2 cytokines if TH-1 cytokines are decreased. In our study the IL-10 production (as a TH-2 cytokine) is decreased (not statistically significant) rather than increased as to be expected regarding this antagonism. Therefore the lower production of IL-2 and IFN-γ in schizophrenic patients is unlikely to be due to this antagonism.

Increased cortisol levels in schizophrenic patients as reported by Ganguli et al. (1993) could not be confirmed by our study. The cortisol levels were found to be normal in all investigated subjects as previously described by Sasaki et al. (1994) and no correlations between IL-2 and cortisol or IFN-γ and cortisol were observed. Serum cortisol levels therefore are probably not responsible for the decreased cytokine production.

Conclusion

In acutely ill schizophrenic patients the production of IFN-γ as well as IL-2 by lymphocytes is impaired. This dysfunction is unlikely to be due to the antagonism between TH-1 and TH-2 cytokines since the production of IL-10 is not increased nor to the serum cortisol levels which were unchanged.

References

Barak V, Barak Y, Levine J, Nisman B, Roisman I (1995) Changes in interleukin-1 beta and soluble interleukin-2 receptor levels in CSF and serum of schizophrenic patients. J Basic Clin Physiol Pharmacol 6:61–69

Becker D, Kritschmann E, Floru S, Shlomo-David Y, Gotlieb-Stematsky T (1990) Serum interferon in first psychotic attack. Br J Psychiatry 157:136–138

Bessler H, Levental Z, Karp L, Modai I, Djaldetti M, Weizman A (1995) Cytokine production in drug-free and neuroleptic-treated schizophrenic patients. Biol Psychiatry 38:297–302

El-Mallakh RS, Suddath RL, Wyatt RJ (1993) Interleukin-1a and interleukin-2 in cerebrospinal fluid of schizophrenic subjects. Prog Neuropsychopharmacol Biol Psychiatry 17:383–391

Ganguli R, Rabin BS (1989) Increased serum interleukin-2 receptor concentration in schizophrenic and brain-damaged subjects. Arch Gen Psychiatry 46:292

Ganguli R, Brar JS, Solomon W, Chengappa KN, Rabin BS (1992) Altered interleukin-2 production in schizophrenia: association between clinical state and autoantibody production. Psychiatry Res 44:113–123

Ganguli R, Brar JS, Chengappa KNR, Yang ZW, Nimgaonkar VL, Rabin BS (1993) Autoimmunity in schizophrenia: a review of recent findings. Ann Med 25:489–496

Ganguli R, Jaspreet SB, Chengappa KNR, DeLeo M, Yang ZW, Shurin G, Rabin BR (1995) Mitogen-stimulated interleukin-2 production in never-medicated first episode schizophrenic patients. Arch Gen Psychiatry 52:668–672

Gattaz WF, Dalgalarrondo P, Schröder HC (1992) Abnormalities in serum concentrations of interleukin-2, interferon-α and interferon-γ in schizophrenia not detected. Schizophr Res 6:237–241

Hornberg M, Arolt V, Wilke I, Kruse A, Kirchner H (1995) Production of interferons and lymphokines in leukocyte cultures of patients with schizophrenia. Schizophr Res 15:237–242

Katila H, Cantell K, Hirvonen S, Rimón R (1989) Production of interferon-α and -γ by leukocytes from patients with schizophrenia. Schizophr Res 2:361–365

Kirch DG (1993) Infection and autoimmunity as etiologic factors in schizophrenia: a review and reappraisal. Schizophr Bull 19:355–370

Kirchner H, Kleinicke C, Digel W (1982) The whole-blood technique for testing production of human interferon by leukocytes. J Immunol Methods 48:213–219

Kita M, Shiozawa S, Yamaji M, Kitoh I, Kishida T (1991) Production of human a- and g-interferon is dependent on age and sex and is decreased in rheumatoid arthritis: a simple method for a large-scale assay. J Clin Lab Anal 5:238–241

Kolyaskina GI (1983) Blood lymphocytes in schizophrenia – immunological and virological aspects. Adv Biol Psychiatry 12:142–149

Kroemer G, Wick G (1989) The role of interleukin 2 in autoimmunity. Immunol Today 10:246–251

Licinio J, Seibyl JP, Altemus M, Charney D, Krystal JH (1993) Elevated CSF levels of interleukin-2 in neuroleptic-free schizophrenic patients. Am J Psychiatry 150: 1408–1410

McAllister CG, van Kammen DP, Rehn TJ, Miller AL, Gurklis J, Kelley ME, Yao J, Peters JL (1995) Increases in CSF levels of interleukin-2 in schizophrenia: effects of recurrence of psychosis and medication status. Am J Psychiatry 152:1291–1297

Moises HW, Schindler L, Leroux M, Kirchner H (1985) Decreased production of interferon alpha and interferon gamma in leukocyte cultures of schizophrenic patients. Acta Psychiatr Scand 72:45–50

Mosmann TR, Moore KW (1991) The role of IL-10 in cross-regulation of TH1 and TH2 responses. Immunoparasitol Today 12:149–153

Preble OT, Torrey EF (1985) Serum interferon in patients with psychosis. Am J Psychiatry 142:1184–1186

Romagnani S (1991) Human TH1 and TH2 subsets: doubt no more. Immunol Today 12:256–257

Romagnani S (1992) Induction of TH1 and TH2 responses: a key role for the "natural" immune response. Immunol Today 13:379–381

Rothermundt M, Arolt V, Weitzsch C, Eckhoff D, Kirchner H (1996) Production of cytokines in acute schizophrenic psychosis. Biol Psychiatry 40:1294–1297

Sasaki T, Nanko S, Fukuda R, Kawate T, Kunugi H, Kazamatsuri H (1994) Changes of immunological functions after acute exacerbation in schizophrenia. Biol Psychiatry 35:173–178

Schindler L, Leroux M, Beck J, Moises HW, Kirchner H (1986) Studies of cellular immunity, serum interferon titers, and natural killer cell activity in schizophrenic patients. Acta Psychiatr Scand 73:651–657

Scott P, Kaufmann SHE (1991) The role of T-cell subsets and cytokines in the regulation of infection. Immunol Today 12:346–348

Syvälahti EKG (1994) Biological factors in schizophrenia. Structural and functional aspects. Br J Psychiatry 164 [Suppl 23]:9–14

Villemain F, Chatenoud L, Galinowski A, Homo-Delarche F, Ginestet D, Loo H, Zarifian E, Bach J-F (1989) Aberrant T cell-mediated immunity in untreated schizophrenic patients: deficient interleukin-2 production. Am J Psychiatry 146: 609–616

Wilke I, Arolt V, Rothermundt M, Weitzsch C, Hornberg M, Kirchner H (1996) Investigations of cytokine production in whole blood cultures of paranoid and residual schizophrenic patients. Eur Arch Psychiatry Clin Neurosci 246:273–278

Wright P, Gill M, Murray RM (1993) Schizophrenia: genetics and the maternal immune response to viral infection. Am J Med Genet 48:40–46

Zlotnik A, Moore KW (1991) Interleukin 10. Cytokine 3:366–371

Correspondence: Dr. M. Rothermundt, Department of Psychiatry, University of Lübeck School of Medicine, Ratzeburger Allee 160, D-23538 Lübeck, Federal Republic of Germany.

Psychoimmunology, anxiety disorders and TMJ-disorders

G. Langs[1], G. Herzog[1], K. Penkner[2], U. Demel[3], G. Tilz[3], R. O. Bratschko[2], and G. Wieselmann[1]

Departments of [1] Psychiatry, [2] Prosthetic Dentistry,
and [3] Immunology, University Hospital, Graz, Austria

Introduction

Stress and anxiety and their relationship to temporo-mandibular-joint (TMJ)-dysfunction pain syndrome has been subject to much research and controversy in recent years. According to Solberg et al. (1981) stress and anxiety lead to an increase of muscle tension in temporo-mandibular muscles. This physiological reaction can result in temporo-mandibular joint pain and dysfunction like occlusional dysfunction, displacement of the disc, bruxism and athrosis (Curran et al., 1996; Jäger et al., 1987; Oakley et al., 1993; Ramfjord, 1961). Therefore stress and anxiety deserve emphasis as a significant underlying cause of TMJ-dysfunction, which has been investigated by a number of studies. Many of them evaluated connections between psychological tests or psychiatric rating scales (e.g. MMPI, Hopkins Symptoms Check List, etc.) on one side, TMJ disorders on the other (Carlson et al., 1993; Stockstill and Callahan, 1991).

There is a high incidence of psychoimmunological alterations in patients suffering from anxiety disorders (Locke et al., 1984; Surmann et al., 1986; Matuzas et al., 1987; Schmidt-Traub, 1991, 1992; Stein et al., 1988; Wieselmann et al., 1995a). However, the mechanism of immunological alterations and anxiety still has not been clarified. The most common hypothesis says that anxiety related stress leads to a suppression of the immune system (Schmidt-Traub, 1991).

The aim of this pilot study was to investigate immunological alterations as well as TMJ-dysfunctions/disorders in patients suffering from anxiety disorders, postulating a possible relationship.

Patients and methods

27 outpatients (7 males mean age 38.6 years, 20 females mean age 36.7 years) were admitted to our anxiety disorders clinic, suffering from panic disorder with (14) or without (13) agoraphobia, according to DSM-III-R criteria (APA, 1987).

Table 1. Grazer dysfunction index

Dysfunction group	points	state of
asymptomatical	< 15	orthofunction
adaptive	15–35	adaptation
adaptive	36–65	compensation
dysfunctional	> 65	malfunction

Table 2. Comparison of panic patients and normal controls

	asymptotical	adaptive (state of adaptation or compensation)
controls	16	10
panic	7	20

Procedures in accordance to Langs et al. (1993):

1. All patients were diagnosed by a physical examination (routine laboratory check, thyroid parameters, ECG), neurological examination and EEG, in order to exclude organic based diseases. To get an exact diagnosis, the psychiatric examination included patient's history, Ham-D as well as standardised interviews (SCID I, DSM-III-R). All patients were drug naive and untreated (no psychotherapy).
2. All patients underwent a proper examination of the TMJ, using the "Grazer dysfunction index" (Riegler and Haas, 1995). This index is computed for patients with functional disorders. It is done by estimating the importance of the relevant epidemiological and symptomatological data of the clinical functional analysis bringing them into relationship. The resultant from the valuation of over 30 parameters is a numerical figure which symbolises a quantitative snap-shot of the functional condition in the stomatognathic system. Using this index prognosis and development of functional disturbances can be assessed. Furthermore, it allows statements concerning the relation between symptoms and individual quality of bioadaptability.
   In order to evaluate the significance of the TMJ-disorders/dysfunctions a sex and age matched control group of 26 healthy volunteers was examined with the "Grazer dysfunction index" too.
3. Furthermore the immune profile consisting of specific and non-specific parameters (autoantibodies / AAB to nuclear factors – ANF / to basement-membrane type 1 and type 2 / to glomerulobasement-membrane – GBM / to ANCA / to DNA / to beta2-microglobuline – Beta2 / to cardiolipin / C-Lip as well as complement levels C3/C4, circulating immune-complexes / CIC=ICOM, soluble interleukin 2-receptors / s-IL2-R=IL2-R, interleukin 2 / IL2, T8, ICAM and gamma-

globuline synthesis / IgA, IgG, IgM) was evaluated and quantitated by indirect immunfluorescence and nephelometry (Tilz et al., 1996).

Results I

All data were compared using χ^2 techniques. There is a significant difference in the frequency of TMJ dysfunctions between anxiety patients and normal controls (χ^2 = 6.292, p > .05, df = 1), as adaptive dysfunctions are more common in panic patients. None of the probands showed a state of malfunction (Table 2).

Results II
Immune profile (18 specific and non-specific parameters)

Immunological alterations are found in the patient sample quite similar to our prior results (Wieselmann et al., 1995b):

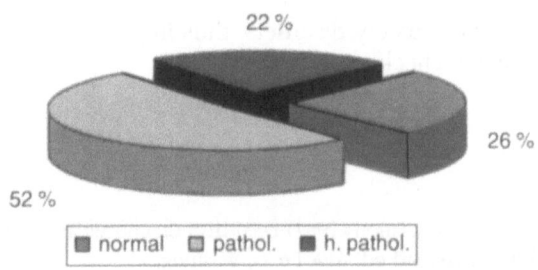

Fig. 1. Immunological alterations I

Conclusion

Chronic stress and anxiety are linked to TMJ-dysfunctions: our results suggest that "anxiety disorders" are actually associated to TMJ-dysfunction and to alterations of the immune system. These retrospective data do not allow to draw any conclusions in which way these disorders and alterations cause each other, but they give further evidence to the hypothesis that somatic changes (Nutt and Lawson, 1992) play an important role in anxiety disorders. These changes may be a matter of vulnerability, maintenance of the disorders or consequence of long-standing psychological stress.

As an outcome of this study the authors emphasise the importance

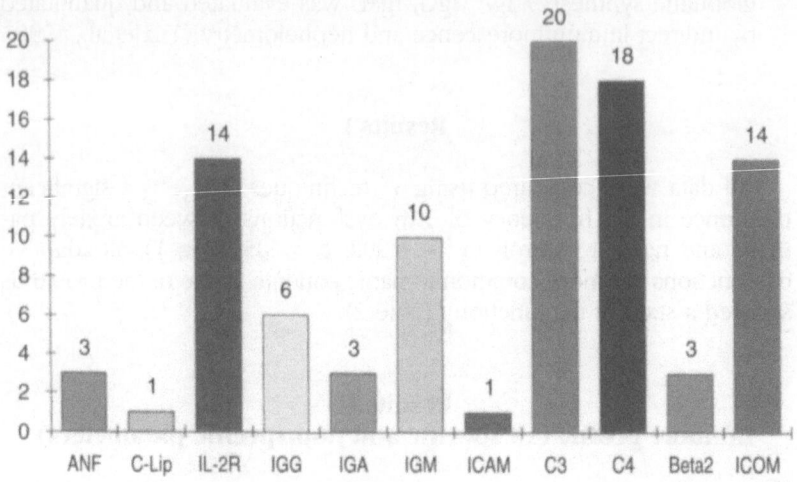

Fig. 2. Immunological alterations II

of a holistic view of anxiety disorders, thus implying the necessity of a thoroughly somatic check up.

References

American Psychiatric Association (1987) DSM III-R diagnostic and statistical manual for mental disorders, 3rd ed. APA Press, Washington

Carlson C, Okeson J, Falace D (1993) Comparison of psychologic and physiologic functioning between patients with masticatory muscle pain and matched controls. J Orofac Pain 7:15–22

Curran SL, Carlson C, Okeson J (1996) Emotional and physiologic responses to laboratory challenges: patients with temporomandibular disorder versus matched control subjects. J Orofac Pain 10:141–149

Jäger K, Borner A, Graber G (1987) Epidemologische Untersuchung über die Ätiologiefaktoren dysfunktioneller Erkrankungen im stomatognathen System. Schweiz Monatsschr Zahnmed 97:1351–1355

Langs G, Wieselmann G, Fabisch H, Melisch B, Fabisch K, Herzog G, Zapotoczky HG (1993) Diagnostisch-therapeutische Konzepte der Panikstörung mit und ohne Agoraphobie. Therapiewoche Österreich 8:643–645

Locke SE, Kraus L, Leserman J, Hurst MW, Heisel JS, Williams RM (1984) Life change stress, psychiatric symptoms, and natural killer cell activity. Psychosom Med 46: 441–453

Matuzas W, Al-Sadir J, Uhlenhuth EH, Glass RN (1987) Mitral valve prolapse and thyroid abnormalities in patients with panic attacks. Am J Psychiatry 144:493–496

Nutt D, Lawson C (1992) Panic attacks. A neurochemical overview of models and mechanisms. Br J Psychiatry 160:165–178

Oakley M, McCreary C, Flack V, Clark G (1993) Screening for psychological problems in TMD-patients. J Orofac Pain 7:143–149

Ramfjord SP (1961) Dysfunctional temporo-mandibular-joint and muscle pain. J Prosthet Dent 11:353

Riegler H, Haas M (1995) Der Grazer Dysfunktionsindex – Eine Methode zur Einschätzung des Funktionszustandes im stomatognathen System. Stomatologie 92: 371–383

Schmidt-Traub S (1991) Angst und immunologische Störung: Phobien, Generalisiertes Angstsyndrom und Panikattacken psychoimmunologisch betrachtet in hypothesengenerierender Absicht. Z Psychol 199:19–34

Schmidt-Traub S, Bamler KJ (1992) Psychoimmunologischer Zusammenhang zwischen Allergien, Panik und Agoraphobien. Z Klin Psychol Psychpathol Psychother 40:325–345

Solberg W, Flint R, Brantner J (1972) Temporomandibular joint pain and dysfunction: a clinical study of emotional and occlusal components. J Prosthet Dent 28:412–422

Stein M, Keller SE, Schleifer SJ (1988) Immune system: relationship to anxiety disorders. Psychiatr Clin North Am 11:349–360

Stockstill J, Callahan C (1991) Personality hardiness, anxiety and depression as constructs of interest in the study of temporomandibular disorder. J Craniomandib Disord, Facial and Oral Pain 5:129–134

Surmann OS, Williams J, Sheehan DV, Strom TB, Jones KJ, Coleman J (1986) Immunological response to stress in agoraphobia and panic attacks. Biol Psychiatry 21:768–774

Tilz G, Faist E, Schreiber F, Demel U, Bäcker H, Demel D, Wachter H, Fuchs D (1996) Soluble interleukin receptor II as a useful tool for diagnosis and treatment of autoimmune infections and malign diseases in clinical medicine and immune pathology: a comparison with other markers of immune activation and therapeutical consequences. In: Faist E (ed) International symposium of shock, trauma and immune diseases. Papst Science Publishers, Berlin, pp 151–154

Wieselmann G, Langs G, Fabisch H, Herzog G, Tilz G, Fabisch K, Demel U (1995a) Immunological investigations in patients suffering from anxiety disorders. Homeostasis 36 [Suppl 1]: 159

Wieselmann G, Langs G, Tilz G, Fabisch H, Herzog G, Fabisch K (1995b) Anxiety disorders: basical measurements, clinical aspects and individual treatment. Behav Pharmacol 6 [Suppl 1]: 41

Correspondence: Dr. G. Langs, Department of Psychiatry, University Hospital, Auenbruggerplatz 22, A-8010 Graz, Austria.

Immunological alterations and neuropsychiatric symptoms: antimicroglia antibodies and psychopathological subgroups in Alzheimer's disease

M. R. Lemke[1], M. Glatzel[2], and A. E. Henneberg[2,3]

[1] Department of Psychiatry, University of Kiel, [2] Department of Neurology, University of Ulm, and [3] Clinic for Parkinson's Disease, Bad Nauheim, Federal Republic of Germany

Introduction

Various immune mechanisms seem to accompany the degenerative process in Alzheimer's disease (AD) and may contribute to the destruction of brain tissue. Acute phase proteins are components of the amyloid of senile plaques and may influence the degradation of amyloid precursor protein into amyloid beta protein (Bauer et al., 1991). Elevation of various cytokines in sera and brain tissue of AD patients and activation of the complement cascade have been demonstrated (Bauer et al., 1992; Aisen and Davis, 1994). Several studies with anti-inflammatory drugs have been reported. However, results are preliminary and not yet conclusive.

Cerebral amyloid deposition seems to occur during an immune-mediated process. Microglia appear to be closely associated with amyloid deposition. Microglia, which may originate as circulating macrophages, are antigen-presenting cells with HLA-DR surface markers (Rogers et al., 1988). The immune process in AD may be a reaction to a foreign antibody or an exposed or altered self-antigen. Therefore, microglia could play an important role in processing the antigen. Antibodies in sera from AD patients directed against cholinergic neuronal CNS structures including hippocampus, cortex and medial septum in rat have been demonstrated. Antibodies directed against microglial cells in vitro were present in cerebrospinal fluid from AD patients (McRae and Dahlström, 1992; McRae et al., 1987, 1991).

AD may not be a homogeneous disease entity and subgroups have been described according to differences in clinical symptomatology and treatment response (Förstl et al., 1994; Lemke, 1995; Mayeux et al., 1985). Diagnostic criteria include cognitive impairment and non-cognitive features including hallucinations, delusions, affective symptoms, behavioral disturbances, and neurological disorders. Behavioral symptoms

Table 1. Main characteristics of Alzheimer's patients and controls

	Alzheimer's patients ($n = 25$)	Controls ($n = 25$)
Age (y)	78.2 ± 8.5	76.8 ± 8.7
	(range 54 to 92)	(range 53 to 92)
Gender	17 m, 8 f	17 m, 8 f
MMSE	6.0 ± 4.0	27.4 ± 1.7
	(range 0 to 13)	(range 25 to 30)

MMSE Mini-Mental-State Examination (Folstein et al., 1975)

including agitation, aggression, motor restlessness, hostility, uncooperativeness, wandering (walking activity, disturbance of diurnal rhythms, faulty goal-directed behavior) rather than cognitive deficits may cause hospitalization or instutionalization. Neuropsychiatric syndroms seem to be related to specific neuroanatomical structures including the limbic system, the amygdala, the hippocampus, and prefrontal cortex (Förstl et al., 1994).

Therefore, sera from AD patients were tested for antibodies directed against human CNS structures (Lemke et al., 1997) and results of antibody binding were correlated with psychopathological symptomatology.

Subjects and methods

Gerontopsychiatric inpatients were included if they fulfilled the following criteria: diagnostic criteria for AD according to DSM-IV (APA, 1994), probable AD according to NINCDS-ADRDA criteria (McKhann et al., 1984), Mini-Mental-State Examination (MMSE) < 16 (Fohlstein et al., 1975). Psychopathological symptoms were rated by the Brief Psychiatric Rating Scale (BPRS). After computing total scores, data of AD patients were analyzed for different BPRS-factor scores including anxiety/depression, anergia, thought, activity, and hostility (Overall and Gorham, 1962).

The following exclusion criteria applied: auto immune diseases, clinical or laboratory signs of acute or chronic infection. The control group comprised inpatients from the department of surgery who showed a MMSE score > 24. Patients with present or past symptoms of psychiatric or immunological disorders or clinical or laboratory signs of acute or chronic infections were excluded. The main characteristics of patients and controls are reported in Table 1.

Blood was drawn by venipuncture between 08.00 and 09.00 a.m., immediately centrifuged and sera were stored at −20 °C. Brain tissue samples were obtained from a 72-year-old patient, who died of embolic lung disease. The patient had no history of psychiatric or immune dis-

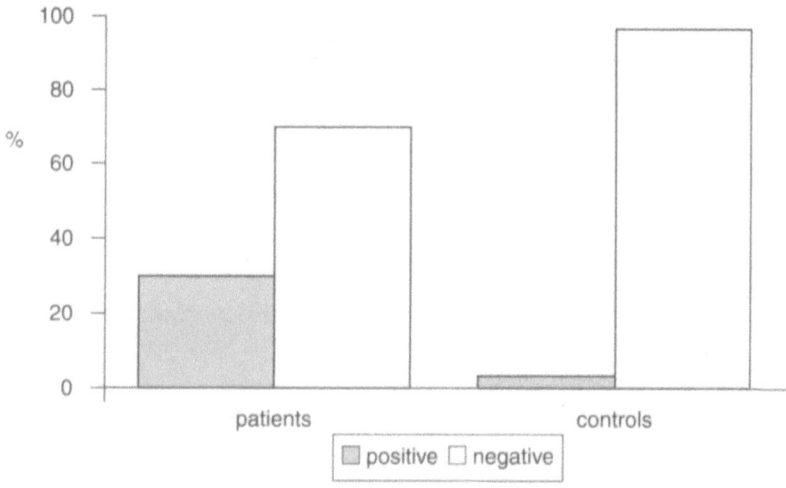

Fig. 1. Binding of antibodies directed against microglia in human post mortem tissue in sera of Alzheimer's patients and control subjects. Significant difference between Alzheimer's patients and control subjects (Fischer's exact test for 2 by 2 tables, two tail, $p = 0.011$)

ease. The brain areas tested did not show any macroscopical or histological changes. Amygdala, frontal and temporal cortex and hippocampus were prepared within 8 hours post mortem. Tissue samples were immediately frozen in liquid nitrogen and stored at −80 °C. The technique of immunofluorescence assay used has been described elsewhere (Henneberg et al., 1993a, b). Patients and their matched controls were tested in a blind fashion at the same day. The samples were recorded as "positive" when specific structures were found that represented anatomical correlates in the histological stain. All samples were evaluated independently by two trained investigators who were in full agreement on the evaluation of the sera as positive or negative.

Results

Antibodies were detected in sera of eight subjects with Alzheimer's disease, whereas only one subject of the control group showed binding to brain tissue (Fig. 1). The specific binding appeared to microglia. The fluorescence seemed to present perinuclear structures of microglial cells. The binding was detected in the IgG- and IgM-compartment. It was mainly directed to nuclei of microglial cells in the amygdala and frontal cortex. Some sera were also positive on temporal cortex and hippocampus (Fig. 2).

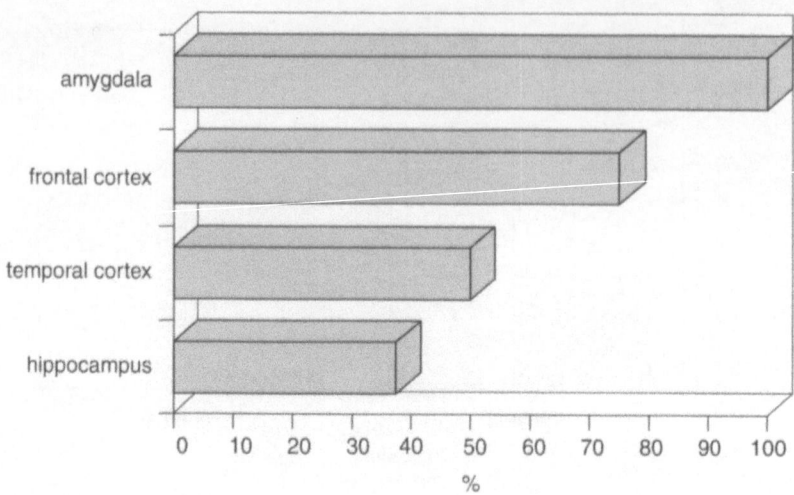

Fig. 2. Areal distribution of antibody binding in sera of positive Alzheimer's disease patients

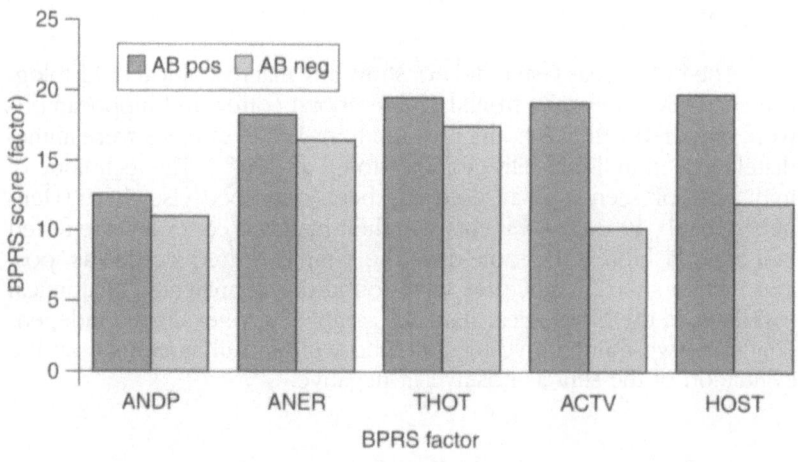

Fig. 3. BPRS-factor scores in AD patients with (AB pos) and without (AB neg) antibody (AB) binding (*ANDP* anxiety/depression, *ANER* anergia, *THOT* thought disturbances, *ACTV* activity, *HOST* hostility)

Patients with and without binding showed no differences in sex or mean age. However, when comparing BPRS scores of patients with positive and negative antibody-binding, significant differences were found in BPRS-factor scores activity and hostility (Fig. 3).

Discussion

There is an extensive amount of literature about immunological alterations which accompany the degenerative process in AD. Acute phase proteins, cytokines and activation of the complement cascade have been demonstrated in brain tissue of AD patients. Preliminary results of treatment studies suggest a therapeutic effect of anti-inflammatory drugs (Aisen and Davis, 1994). Antibodies in sera of AD patients directed against cholinergic neuronal CNS structures of the rat have been demonstrated. Antibodies directed against microglial cells in vitro were shown in cerebrospinal fluid from AD patients (McRae and Dahlström, 1992). Because most studies showed antibody binding to rat CNS or in in vitro models, this study was carried out to detect antibodies in sera of AD patients directed against human post mortem tissue. Brain areas that have been postulated to be affected in AD were chosen. The immunofluorescence method used meets the recommendations of the WHO for searching autoantibodies (Thompson, 1988). All experiments were carried out in a well-controlled way including blinded investigators for diagnosis and testing patients and controls in coded samples on the same day.

Approximately one third of the AD patients, but only one subject of the control group, showed IgG- and IgM-binding to the nuclei of microglial cells. All patients were diagnosed according to NINCDS-ADRDA criteria for probable AD. However, diagnosis of definite AD can only be confirmed by biopsy or autopsy. AD may not be a homogeneous disease entity and subgroups have been described according to differences in clinical symptomatology (Mayeux et al., 1985) and treatment response (Lemke, 1995). Thus, patients with anti-microglia antibodies may represent a biologically defined subgroup of AD in which immune mechanisms may play a role in the etiology of the disease (Lemke et al., 1997).

The fact that one control serum showed binding to microglia may be explained by findings in other autoimmune disorders. A twin study in myasthenia gravis showed autoantibodies to acetylcholine receptors also in the non-affected twin (Lefvert et al., 1989). Thus, autoantibodies without clinical manifestation may not exclude the presence of an autoimmune disorder. Clinical follow up of the positive control subject is necessary. Because patients and controls were closely age matched, age linked phenomena can be excluded. Due to multimorbidity, most patients in the study received various medications including neuroleptics, carbamazepine, benzodiazepines and others. Medication effects can not be excluded. However, using this test system in schizophrenic patients, no influence of neuroleptic medication was detected (Henneberg et al., 1993b).

Antibodies directed against microglia may be an early marker of a neurodegenerative process before clinical manifestations. The relationship between the course of the disease and the presence of antibodies needs further evaluation. Cerebral amyloid deposition seems to occur during immune mediated processes (Bauer et al., 1991, 1992). An unknown pathogen (trauma, cell death and others) may stimulate microglia to produce interleukin-6, which in turn induces alpha-2-macroglobulin, which could impair the processing of the amyloid precursor protein, giving rise to the pathogenic beta-A4-molecule, which aggregates to participate in plaque formation. This abnormal molecule could be presented to T-cells, which extravate from CNS, activate B-cells and antibody production (McRae and Dahlström, 1992). Thus, novel treatment strategies involving immunotherapy may be effective in delaying or reversing the progression of neurodegeneration.

AD patients with positive antibody binding showed higher scores in behavioral symptoms including activity and hostility. Because AD may not be a homogeneous disease entity, subgroups have been described according to differences in clinical symptomatology and treatment response (Förstl et al., 1994; Lemke, 1995; Mayeux et al., 1985). Diagnostic criteria include cognitive impairment and non-cognitive features including hallucinations, delusions, affective symptoms, behavioral disturbances and neurological disorders. Behavioral symptoms including agitation, aggression, motor restlessness, hostility, uncooperativeness, wandering (walking activity, disturbance of diurnal rhythms, faulty goal-directed behavior) rather than cognitive deficits may cause hospitalization or instutionalization. Neuropsychiatric syndroms may be related to specific neuroanatomical structures including the limbic system, the amygdala, the hippocampus, and prefrontal cortex (Förstl et al., 1994). In the AD patients studied, no difference in severity of cognitive impairment was found between patients with or without antibody binding. However, patients with positive antibody binding displayed more behavioral disturbances including activity and hostility. These neuropsychiatric symptoms may be related to limbic structures including the amygdala. The medial nucleus of the amygdala has been implicated to play a role in regulation of activity and aggression. Because all patients showed positive antibody binding directed against structures of the amygdala, the results may indicate a connection between immunological reactions, neuroanatomical structures and neuropsychiatric symptoms. More work needs to be done to test this hypothesis.

In conclusion, anti-microglial antibodies can be detected in a subgroup of AD patients suggesting involvement of immunological mechanisms in these patients. Further studies are necessary to evaluate the relationship with course, severity, and clinical subgroups of the disease. Positive antibody binding in the amygdala may be related to neuropsychiatric symptoms. The findings warrant further studies to test the hypothesis of specific immunological reactions underlying neuropsychiatric symptoms and disorders.

References

Aisen PS, Davis KL (1994) Inflammatory mechanisms in Alzheimer's disease: implication for therapy. Am J Psychiatry 151:1105–1113

American Psychiatric Association (1994) Diagnostic and statistical manual, 4th edn (DSM-IV). APA, Washington DC

Bauer J, Strauss S, Schreiter-Gasser U, Ganter U, Schlegel P, Witt I, Volk B, Berger M (1991) Interleukin-6 and alpha-2-macroglobulin indicate an acute phase response in Alzheimer's disease cortices. FEBS Lett 285:111–114

Bauer J, Ganter U, Strauss S, Stadtmüller G, Frommberger U, Bauer H, Volk B, Berger M (1992) The participation of interleukin-6 in the pathogenesis of Alzheimer's disease. Res Immunol 143:650–657

Folstein MF, Folstein SE, McHugh PR (1975) "Mini-Mental State": a practical method for grading the cognitive state of patients for the clinician. J Psychiatr Res 12: 189–198

Förstl H, Burns A, Levy P, Cairns N (1994) Neuropathological correlates of psychotic phenomena in confirmed Alzheimer's disease. Br J Psychiatry 165:53–59

Henneberg AE, Ruffert S, Henneberg H-J, Kornhuber HH (1993a) Antibodies to brain tissue in sera of schizophrenic patients – preliminary findings. Eur Arch Psychiatry Clin Neurosci 242:314–317

Henneberg AE, Yueksektepeli B, Bauer M (1993b) Brain antibodies in sera of patients suffering from schizophrenia or schizoaffective diseases, but not from neurotic disorders: the phenomenon is independent from medication. Immunobiol 189: 220–221

Lemke MR (1995) Effect of carbamazepine on agitation in Alzheimer's inpatients refractory to neuroleptics. J Clin Psychiatry 56:354–357

Lemke MR, Glatzel M, Henneberg AE (1997) Anti-microglia antibodies in sera of Alzheimer's disease patients. Biol Psychiatry (in press)

Mayeux P, Stern Y, Spanton S (1985) Heterogeneity in dementia of the Alzheimer type: evidence of subgroups. Neurology 35:453–461

McKhann G, Drachman D, Folstein M, Katzman R, Peice D, Stadlan E (1984) Clinical diagnosis of Alzheimer's disease: report of the NINCDS-ARDA work group under the auspices of the Department of Health and Human Services Task Force on Alzheimer's Disease. Neurology 34:939–944

McRae A, Dahlström A (1992) Cerebrospinal fluid antibodies: an indicator for immune responses in Alzheimer's disease. Res Immunol 143:663–667

McRae A, Ling EA, Polinsky P, Gottfries CG, Dahlström A (1991) Antibodies in the cerebrospinal fluid from some Alzheimer's disease patients recognize amoeboid microglial cells in the developing rat central nervous system. Neuroscience 41: 739–752

McRae-Dagueurce A, Bööj S, Haglig K, Rosengren L, Karsson JE, Karlsson I, Wallin A, Svennerholm L, Gottfries CG, Dahlström A (1987) Antibodies in the cerebrospinal fluid of some Alzheimer's disease patients recognize cholinergic neurons in the rat central nervous system. Proc Acad Sci (Wash) 84:9214–9218

Overall JE, Gorham DR (1962) The brief psychiatric rating scale. Psychol Rep 10: 799–812

Rogers J, Luber-Narod J, Styren SD, Civin WH (1988) Expression of immune system-associated antigen by cells of the human central nervous system: relationship to the pathology of Alzheimer disease. Neurobiol Aging 9:330–349

Thompson RA (1988) Laboratory investigations in clinical immunology: methods, pitfalls and clinical indications. Clin Exp Immunol 74:494–503

Correspondence: M. R. Lemke, M. D., Department of Psychiatry, University of Kiel, Niemannsweg 147, D-24105 Kiel, Federal Republic of Germany.

Platelet antibodies in mental disorder

K. Schott[1], M. Schnaidt[2], A. Batra[1], M. Bartels[1], and G. Buchkremer[1]

[1] Universitätsklinik für Psychiatrie und Psychotherapie and [2] Abteilung für Transfusionsmedizin, Tübingen, Federal Republic of Germany

Introduction

Platelets are a model for monoamine containing neurons in the CNS (Sneddon, 1973; Pletcher et al., 1984). Serotonin and dopamine uptake mechanisms are well established in this model (Lingjaerde, 1977; Gordon and Overman, 1978; Omenn and Smith, 1978; Lingjaerde and Kildemo, 1981). Shinitzky and co-workers (1991) first demonstrated platelet associated antibodies (PAA) in schizophrenia and dementia which cross-reacted with brain tissue from rats. Kessler and Shinitzky (1993) showed that PAA from schizophrenic patients specifically inhibited the uptake of dopamine by platelets and interfered with the dopamine receptor ligands [3H]-dopamine and [3H]-spiperone at rat brain P2m membranes. The authors suggested that blood platelets may function as a peripheral epitope for the formation of PAA, which, when reaching the brain, may react with the dopamine receptor and elicit mental disorder. In this context alterations of the immune status with occurrence of autoantibodies in schizophrenia are known for decades (Brauchitsch, 1972; DeLisi et al., 1985; Stein et al., 1987). In this study we investigated the formation of anti platelet antibodies in patients with various mental disorders.

Methods

Subjects. All patients and healthy controls gave their informal consent to the study. Healthy controls and patients are further characterized in Table 1 as to sex, age, duration of illness, number of episodes, and medication. Controls were healthy blood donors. The psychiatric patients were diagnosed according to RDC (Spitzer et al., 1978).

Blood samples were obtained at routine venipuncture between 7:00 and 9:00 a. m. and the serum frozen at $-30\,°C$ until analysis.

Screening for platelet antibodies. Screening for platelet reactive IgG and IgM serum antibodies was done by a platelet-immunofluorescence-test (PIFT). EDTA was added to all samples in a final concentration of

Table 1. Characterization of controls and patients

Diagnosis	Sex	N	age		duration (ys)		episodes		medication	
			median	range	median	range	median	range	TCA	NLP
controls	m	10	24.5	22–64						
	f	10	25.5	21–52						
MD	m	6	55.5	24–75	2	1–55	2.5	2–6	6	4
	f	14	60.5	35–75	7	1–40	2.5	1–5	13	11
PS	m	8	32	23–49	4.5	0–19	1	1–3	3	5
	f	12	33	21–52	8.5	3–29	4	3–4	6	12
SAP	m	9	33.5	24–54	13	0–28	3	1–11	6	9
	f	11	39.5	24–56	7	1–36	4	2–18	8	11
ALC	m	13	38	27–59	9	1–29			5	7
	f	7	43	33–70	6	1–20			2	3

MD major depression; *PS* paranoid schizophrenia; *SAP* schizoaffective psychosis; *ALC* alcoholism; *TCA* tricyclic antidepressants; *NLP* neuroleptics; *m* male; *f* female

Table 2. Platelet antibodies

Diagnosis	N	IgM pos.	IgG pos.
controls	20	10 %	5 %
MD	20	5 %	0 %
PS	20	45 %	0 %
SAP	20	15 %	15 %
ALC	20	50 %	5 %

MD major depression; *PS* paranoid schizophrenia; *SAP* schizoaffective psychosis; *ALC* alcoholism

0.3% (w/v) thus demonstrating EDTA-dependent platelet antibodies in addition to other platelet reactive auto- or alloantibodies. All sera showing positive results in this screening were investigated further in PIFT without EDTA and in the MAIPA-assay (a glycoprotein specific ELISA) in order to characterize EDTA-dependent antibodies, platelet specific auto- or alloantibodies and HLA-antibodies. The PIFT was performed in a modification described by Schneider and Schnaidt (1981) using platelets of two donors of blood group 0. For antibody detection FITC-conjugated anti IgG and IgM antibodies (DAKO, Denmark) were used. The MAIPA-assay (monoclonal-antibody-specific immobilization of platelet antigens, Kiefel et al., 1987) in the modifications described by Kiefel et al. (1994) was performed using monoclonal antibodies directed to glycoprotein complex (GP) IIb/IIIa (P2, Dianova), GP Ib/IX (SZ1, Dianova) and β2-microglobulin (B1G6, Dianova). Bound antibodies were visualized with peroxidase-conjugated antihuman IgG and IgM antibodies. As test cells platelets from the same donors as in the PIFT were used.

Statistical analysis. Data were evaluated statistically by Fisher's exact test.

Results

The results with regard to EDTA-dependent platelet antibodies in PIFT are listed in Table 2.

About 45% of patients with paranoid schizophrenia ($p < 0.05$) and 50% of patients with alcoholism ($p < 0.01$) were positive for anti platelet IgM antibodies. Healthy controls showed IgM antibodies in 10% and IgG antibodies in 5% only. The results of the two other test groups were not significant.

With regard to the MAIPA-assay the following results were obtained. In healthy controls two persons were positive for GP IIb/IIIa and one person for GP Ib/IX. In patients with major depression two persons were positive for GP IIb/IIIa and one person for GP Ib/IX. In patients with paranoid schizophrenia one person was positive for GP IIb/IIIa

and GP Ib/IX. In schizoaffective psychosis one person was positive for
GP IIb/IIIa. In chronic alcoholism nobody was positive for GP antigens.

Discussion

Alterations of the immune status in schizophrenia are well known
(DeLisi et al., 1985; Stein et al., 1987). The occurrence of brain reactive
autoantibodies in this disorder was interpreted on the basis of an underlying autoimmune process of the brain. The existence of CNS specific
antigen–antibody systems with antibodies directed to important target
molecules of the brain could explain the pathological impact of brain
reactive autoantibodies on the development of mental disorder. In this
context platelets are a model for monoamine containing neurons in the
CNS (Sneddon, 1973; Pletcher et al., 1984) and platelet associated antibodies (PAA) were shown to bind to rat brain (Shinitzky et al., 1991) and
to interfere with dopamine ligands at the dopamine receptor (Kessler
and Shinitzky, 1993). Therefore, we investigated the formation of anti
platelet antibodies in patients with various mental disorders. The most
important finding was the proof of EDTA dependent IgM antibodies in
paranoid schizophrenia (45%) and alcoholism (50%). Healthy controls
were positive in 10%. We interpreted these results on the basis of the
known effects of PAA on neurotransmission. At least in a subgroup of
patients with paranoid schizophrenia platelet antibodies may indicate
an autoimmune process with possible implications for the dopaminergic neurotransmission. To our surprise patients with chronic alcoholism
were highly positive as well (50%). Also in this case an autoimmune process appears to play a role in the pathogenesis of the disease. The trigger
for antibody production is unknown and may arise in response to an
unrelated antigen, and the antibody may then cross-react with platelets.
Only few sera were positive for glycoprotein complex antigens of platelet membranes which play a role in acute and chronic autoimmune
thrombocytopenia. Thus the autoimmune process in paranoid schizophrenia and alcoholism follows a different pathway. In summary there
is some evidence of an autoimmune process with occurrence of platelet
antibodies in paranoid schizophrenia and alcoholism which may have a
pathological impact on the dopaminergic neurotransmission in the brain.

References

Brauchitsch H (1972) Antinuclear factor in psychiatric disorders. Am J Psychiatry
    128:1552–1554
DeLisi LE, Weber RJ, Pert CB (1985) Are there antibodies against brain in sera from
    schizophrenic patients? Review and prospectus. Biol Psychiatry 20:94–119

Gordon JL, Overman HJ (1978) Hydroxytryptamine and dopamine transport by rat and human platelets. Br J Pharmacol 62:219–226

Kessler A, Shinitzky M (1993) Platelets from schizophrenic patients bear autoimmune antibodies that inhibit dopamine uptake. Psychobiology 21:299–306

Kiefel V, Santoso S, Weisheit M, Mueller-Eckhardt C (1987) Monoclonal antibody specific immobilization of platelet antigens (MAIPA): a new tool for the identification of platelet reactive antibodies. Blood 70:1722–1726

Kiefel V, Scheld S, Freitag E, Kroll H, Mueller-Eckhardt C (1994) Zwei Modifikationen des MAIPA-Assays zum Nachweis thrombozytärer Antikörper. In: Sibrowski W, Stangel W, Wegener S (eds) Transfusionsmedizin 1993/94. Beitr Infusionsther Transfusionsmed, vol 32. Karger, Basel, pp 237–239

Lingjaerde O (1977) Platelet uptake and storage of serotonin. In: Essan EW (ed) Serotonin in health and disease. Spectrum, New York, pp 129–199

Lingjaerde O, Kildemo O (1981) Dopamine uptake in platelets: two different low affinity saturable mechanisms. Agents & Actions 11:410–416

Omenn GS, Smith LT (1978) A common uptake system for serotonin and dopamine in human platelets. J Clin Invest 58:235–240

Pletcher A, Affolter H, Cesuka M, Erne E, Mueller K (1984) Blood platelets as models for neurons: similarities of the 5-hydroxy-tryptamine systems. In: Schlossberger HG, Kochen W, Linzen B, Steinhart H (eds) Progress in tryptophan and serotonin research. De Gruyter, Berlin, pp 231–239

Schneider W, Schnaidt M (1981) The platelet adhesion immunofluorescence test: a modification of the platelet suspension immunofluorescence test. Blut 43:389–392

Shinitzky M, Deckmann M, Kessler A, Sirota P, Rabbs A, Elizur A (1991) Platelet autoantibodies in dementia and schizophrenia. Ann NY Acad Sci 621:205–217

Sneddon M (1973) Blood platelets as a model for monoamine containing neurons. In: Kerkut GA, Phillips JW (eds) Progress in neurobiology. Pergamon, New York, pp 151–192

Spitzer RL, Endicott J, Robins E (1978) Research diagnostic criteria. Arch Gen Psychiatry 35:773–782

Stein M, Schleifer SJ, Keller SE (1987) Brain, behavior, and immune processes. In: Michels R, Cavenar JO, Brody HKH, Cooper AM, Guze SB, Judd LL, Klerman GL, Solnit AJ (eds) Psychiatry, 2nd rev ed, vol 2. Basic Books Inc, New York, pp 1–19

Correspondence: Dr. K. Schott, Universitätsklinik für Psychiatrie und Psychotherapie, Osianderstrasse 24, D-72076 Tübingen, Federal Republic of Germany.

Plasma levels of interleukin 1β and interleukin 6 in mental disorders

K. Schott, A. Batra, A. Uhl, M. Bartels, and G. Buchkremer

Psychiatrische Universitätsklinik, Tübingen, Federal Republic of Germany

Introduction

It was concluded from alterations of interleukins in CSF and plasma that patients with schizophrenia and major depression exhibit an acute stimulation of the immune system [1, 2, 3, 4]. In this context an underlying autoimmune process was assumed in the pathology of schizophrenia and major depression. Especially schizophrenia with its relapsing and chronic forms reminds of the course of autoimmune diseases like chronic rheumatic illness [5, 6].

Not only stimulation of interleukins and cellular subsets of lymphocytes point to an involvement of the immune system but also humoral factors with stimulated antibodies against brain proteins [7, 8], neuropeptides (9), neurotransmitters [10], and antinuclear antibodies [11, 12]. Nevertheless, the investigations were contradictory to a large extent [13, 14, 15, 16]. Findings with significant results faced studies with negative results. This may be due to heterogenous groups of schizophrenic and depressed patients as well as to methodological differences of the various studies. As regards the results of the interleukin investigations almost all authors claimed an increase of interleukin 1α, interleukin 1β, interleukin 2, and interleukin 6 in plasma or in vitro after mitogenic stimulation of lympholyts from patients with schizophrenia and major depression [1, 2, 3, 4, 17, 18, 19, 20].

A few authors did not find any difference to controls [21]. In this study we investigated plasma levels of interleukin 1β and interleukin 6 from patients with paranoid schizophrenia and major depression by an ELISA method.

Material and methods

Up to 41 healthy volunteers and patients with paranoid schizophrenia and major depression participated in the study. A further characterization as to number, sex, and age is compiled in Tables 1 and 2. All patients had a medication with neuroleptics or tricyclic antidepressants.

Table 1. Interleukin-1β-measurement: characterization of test groups

Diagnosis	n	Sex		Age	
		male	female	mean	range
Major depression	7	1	6	61.1	46–71
Paranoid schizophrenia	18	11	7	33.1	20–51
Controls	16	6	10	37.6	26–56

Table 2. Interleukin-6-measurement: characterization of test groups

Diagnosis	n	Sex		Age	
		male	female	mean	range
Major depression	7	1	6	61.1	46–71
Paranoid schizophrenia	16	10	6	33.6	20–51
Controls	16	6	10	38.1	26–56

The patients were diagnosed according to RDC [22]. Blood samples were collected at routine venipuncture from 07.00 to 08.00 a. m. and the plasma stored at −20 °C until analysis.

ELISA test systems for detection of interleukin 1β and interleukin 6 in plasma were purchased from Dianova (Hamburg).

Results and discussion

The results of the interleukin investigations are summarized in Tables 3 and 4. In the case of interleukin 1β only one patient with major depression out of 7 (14.3%) showed a significant elevation of interleukin 1β in plasma. As regards interleukin 6 again only one patient with major depression was above controls. Thus we could not confirm earlier studies claiming an increase of interleukins in mental disorder. Our view is supported by a recent study from Katila et al. [21] who reported unchanged interleukin levels in the plasma of schizophrenic patients either. Xu et al. [23] showed that elevated concentrations of interleukin 1α and interleukin 6 were due to the neuroleptic medication in schizophrenic patients. The difference of results in all these studies remains unclear at last. One could speculate that differences in methodology and recruitment of patients may play a role. Another problem is that the concentrations of interleukins in plasma are low and do not automatically represent the immunological state of an organism. Furthermore, in mental disorder one would expect an immunological dysregulation in the central nervous system. Therefore the present literature findings on alterations of interleukins in plasma do not allow for an unequivocal statement in favor of an autoimmune process in mental disorders.

Table 3. Interleukin-1β-measurement: frequency of pathologically elevated plasma specimens

Diagnosis	n	positive %
Major depression	7	14.3
Paranoid schizophrenia	18	0
Controls	16	18.8

Table 4. Interleukin-6-measurement: frequency of pathologically elevated plasma specimens

Diagnosis	n	positive %
Major depression	7	14.3
Paranoid schizophrenia	16	0
Controls	16	0

Acknowledgements

This study was supported by a grant from the Volkswagen Foundation (I 68 248).

References

[1] Ganguli R, McAllister CG, Rabin BS, Solomon W, Brar JS, Rehn I (1991) Alterations in interleukins and in lymphocyte subsets in a subgroup of schizophrenia. Biol Psychiatry 29:109 A

[2] Shintani F, Kanba S, Marno N, Nakaki T, Nibuya M, Suzuki E, Kinoshita N, Yagi G (1991) Serum interleukin 6 in schizophrenic patients. Life Sci 49:661–664

[3] Licinio J, Seibyl JP, Altemus M, Charney DS, Krystal JH (1993) Elevated CSF levels of interleukin-2 in neuroleptic free schizophrenic patients. Am J Psychiatry 150: 1408–1410

[4] Maes M, Stevens WJ, Declerck LS, Bridts CH, Peeters D, Schotte G, Cosyns P (1993) Significantly increased expression of T-cell activation markers (Interleukin-2 and HAL-DR) in depression. Further evidence for an inflammatory process during that illness. Progr Neuropsychopharmacol Biol Psychiatry 17:241–255

[5] Knight J, Knight A, Ungvari G (1992) Can autoimmune mechanisms account for the genetic predisposition to schizophrenia? Br J Psychiatry 160:533–540

[6] DeLisi LE, Weber RJ, Pert CB (1985) Are there antibodies against brain in sera from schizophrenic patients? Review and prospectus. Biol Psychiatry 20:94–119

[7] Ganguli R, Rabin BS, Kelly RH, Lyte M, Ragu U (1987) Clinical and laboratory evidence of autoimmunity in acute schizophrenia. Ann NY Acad Sci 496:676–685

[8] Heath RG, McCarron KL, O'Neil CE (1989) Antiseptal brain antibody in IgG of schizophrenic patients. Biol Psychiatry 25:725–733

[9] Roy BF, Rose JW, Sunderland T, Morihsa JM, Murphy DL (1988) Antisomatostatin IgG in major depressive disorder. Arch Gen Psychiatry 45:924–928

[10] Schott K, Batra A, Klein R, Bartels M, Koch W, Berg PA (1992) Antibodies against serotonin and gangliosides in schizophrenia and major depressive disorder. Eur Psychiatry 7:209–212

[11] Brauchitsch H (1972) Antinuclear factor in psychiatric disorders. Am J Psychiatry 128:1552–1554

[12] Sirota P, Firer MA, Schild K, Tanay A, Elizur A, Meytes D, Slor H (1993) Auto-

antibodies to DNA in multi case families with schizophrenia. Biol Psychiatry 33: 450–455

[13] Ehrnst A, Wiesel FA, Bjerkenstedt LB, Tribukait B, Jonsson J (1982) Failure to detect immunological stigmata in schizophrenia. Neuropsychobiol 8:169–171

[14] Knight JG, Knight A, Menkes DB, Mullen PE (1990) Autoantibodies against brain septal region antigens specific to unmedicated schizophrenia? Biol Psychiatry 28: 467–474

[15] Fontana A, Storck U, Angst J, Dubs R, Abegg A, Grob PJ (1980) An immunological basis of schizophrenia and affective disorders? Neuropsychobiol 6:284–289

[16] Whalley LJ, Roberts DF, Wentzel J, Watson KL (1981) Antinuclear antibodies and histocompatibility antigens in patients on long-term lithium therapy. J Affect Disord 3:123–130

[17] Maes M, Bosmans E, Meltzer HY, Scharpe S, Suy E (1993) Interleukin-1β: a putative mediator of HPA axis hyperactivity in major depression. Am J Psychiatry 150:1189–1193

[18] Rapaport MH, Torrey EF, McAllister CG, Nelson DL, Pickar D, Paul SM (1993) Increased serum soluble interleukin 2-receptors in schizophrenic monozygotic twins. Eur Arch Psychiatry Clin Neurosci 243:7–10

[19] Yang ZLO, Chengappa KNR, Shurin G, Brar JS, Rabin BS, Gubbi AN, Ganguli R (1994) An association between anti-hipocampal antibody concentration and lymphocyte production of Il-2 in patients with schizophrenia. Psychol Med 24: 449–455

[20] Maes M, Meltzer HY, Buckley P, Bosmans E (1995) Plasma soluble interleukin-2 and transferin receptor in schizophrenia and major depression. Eur Arch Psychiatry Clin Neurosci 244:325–329

[21] Katila H, Hurme M, Wahlbeck K, Appelberg B, Rimond R (1994) Plasma and cerebrospinal fluid interleukin-1β and interleukin-6 in hospitalized schizophrenic patients. Neuropsychobiol 30:20–30

[22] Spitzer RL, Endicott J, Robins E (1978) Research diagnostic criteria. Arch Gen Psychiatry 35:773–782

[23] Xu HM, Wie J, Hemmings GB (1994) Changes of plasma concentrations of interleukin-1α and interleukin-6 with neuroleptic treatment for schizophrenia. Br J Psychiatry 164:251–253

Correspondence: Dr. K. Schott, Psychiatrische Universitätsklinik, Osianderstrasse 24, D-72076 Tübingen, Federal Republic of Germany.

Effects of cytokines on human EEG and sleep

J. Born[1] and E. Späth-Schwalbe[2]

[1] Department of Clinical Neuroendocrinology, University of Luebeck, and Department of Physiological Psychology, University of Bamberg, and
[2] Department of Internal Medicine, Humboldt University, Charité, Berlin, Federal Republic of Germany

Introduction

Numerous experiments in animals have indicated a mutual interdependency between central nervous sleep/wake processes and immunological functions (Krüger et al., 1990; Krüger and Karnovsky, 1995; Toth, 1995). Two principally different concepts have guided this research. On the one hand, it was assumed that sleep has a general restoring effect, and in this context also facilitates immune functioning (e.g., Dinges et al., 1994; Born et al., 1997). On the other hand, the hypothesis has been put forward that the immune system influences sleep. Support for this latter view derived from common observations that infectious diseases may be accompanied by intense feelings of tiredness and sleepiness. Immune processes may induce and maintain central nervous sleep via the release of cytokines which are the messengers of the immune system. In animals, especially cytokines initiating the immune response such as the monocyte/macrophage derived cytokines tumor necrosis factor-α (TNF-α) and interleukin-1 (IL-1) but also interferons (IFNs) have been shown to facilitate sleep (e.g., Shoham et al., 1987; Krüger et al., 1984, 1987, 1990). This paper concentrates on studies examining whether proinflammatory cytokines exert a similar promoting effect on human sleep.

This question is also of potential relevance for the understanding of psychopathology. A very common symptom of various psychiatric diseases is the severe disturbance of sleep. In subgroups of these patients, the sleep disturbancies appear to coincide with distinct immune alterations which, indeed, could be the cause for the alterations of sleep (e.g., Appelberg et al., 1997; Ganguli et al., 1993). However, the hypothesis that cytokines could be regulators of sleep, so far, has been examined primarily in animal experiments in which these cytokines were administered. In humans, the effects of cytokines on electroencephalographic (EEG) activity and sleep, so far, have been tested only in a few clinical trials (Mattson et al., 1983, 1987; Born et al., 1989). To the best of our knowledge, in healthy humans only one study has been conducted examining effects of IL-6 (Späth-Schwalbe et al., 1996). This is in part due to the fact that many of these substances have become available for the use in humans only recently.

Clinical trials in patients

First attempts to study effects of cytokines on human EEG activity and sleep have been undertaken in clinical trials with cancer patients who were treated with these substances as part of their therapy. As an example of this approach, a study is illustrated which aimed to assess effects of IFN-α and IFN-γ in patients with hairy cell leucemia and other types of neoplastic diseases in a metastatic state including thyroid cancer, renal cancer, neurosarcoma and adrenocortical carcinoma (Born et al., 1989). These patients were treated subchronically with high doses of IFN-α (between 1.5×10^6 and 3×10^6 IU) or IFN-γ (between 3.4×10^6 and 30×10^6 IU) administered between 1 and 5 times per week. Following a pretreatment baseline session each patient was tested at least two times during treatment with IFN. IFN was injected subcutaneously at 9.00 h, and test sessions took place between 1200 and 1600 h, on the first day of the IFN treatment and then once every week on days of IFN administration. On each session, spontaneous EEG recordings during rest (with closed eyes) were obtained. Resting EEG activity was analysed after Fast Fourier Transformation with respect to the power within different frequency bands. In addition to spontaneous EEG activity, standard recordings of auditory and visual evoked brain potential responses were obtained. From twelve patients initially included in the study, 3 had to be excluded because IFN treatment was followed by high fever which prevented timely testing.

In general, effects of IFN on EEG activity did not appear to differ in quality between the second session (i.e., on the first day of IFN treatment) and third session (i.e., after one week of IFN treatment). But the effects were more pronounced with prolonged treatment. Also, there was no clear evidence for differential central nervous effects of IFN-γ and IFN-α, although the number of patients treated with IFN-α ($n = 3$) was too small to allow for solid conclusions. Table 1 compares results from the pretreatment baseline session and from the third session after one week of IFN treatment.

Both IFNs reduced power within the α-frequency band (7–14 Hz) and also within the β-frequency band (14–26 Hz) with this effect reaching significance after one week of treatment with IFN. Power within the slower theta frequency band was not affected by IFN treatment. These results suggested an increased cortical excitability during therapy with IFNs, a view which was also supported by findings on evoked

Table 1. Mean power density for the θ, α and β frequencies of the spontaneous EEG activity, latencies of the major components of the visual evoked potential (VEP: N80, P100) and the brainstem auditory evoked potential (BAEP: V, Vn)

Parameter	Baseline	IFN		
	mean ± SEM	mean ± SEM	Difference vs. baseline	
	across IFN-γ and IFN-α		IFN-γ	IFN-α
EEG mean power density, μV^2/Hz				
θ (3–7 Hz)	3.076 ± 0.52	3.434 ± 0.79	+0.603	−0.375
α (7–14 Hz)	5.202 ± 1.49	3.255 ± 0.58**	−2.440*	−0.456
β (14–26 Hz)	0.933 ± 0.17	0.560 ± 0.10**	−0.430**	−0.200
VEP latencies, ms				
N80	76.95 ± 2.37	75.50 ± 2.13	−1.40	−1.40
P100	110.25 ± 1.54	105.40 ± 2.82**	−6.60**	−1.45
BAEP latencies, ms				
V (80 dB HL)	5.66 ± 0.10	5.54 ± 0.09	−0.14*	−0.04
V (40 dB HL)	7.01 ± 0.26	6.99 ± 0.26	0.09	−0.70
V_n (80 dB HL)	6.57 ± 0.12	6.49 ± 0.11*	−0.11*	−0.03
V_n (40 dB HL)	8.20 ± 0.24	7.88 ± 0.23**	−0.37**	−0.05
Temperature, °C	37.0 ± 0.16	37.6 ± 0.26**	+1.0**	−0.3

Means ± SEM (across patients treated with IFN-γ or α) are indicated for the baseline session and the second session during IFN therapy (i.e., after one week of IFN treatment). In addition, the mean differences from the baseline are indicated separately for patients treated with IFN-γ ($n = 6$) or IFN-α ($n = 3$; column "Difference vs. baseline"). VEPs were recorded to checkerboard reversals (rate 1.1/s). BAEPs were recorded to clicks of 80 and 40 dB HL intensity (click rate 10/s). Significant differences from baseline values are indicated with ** $p < 0.05$ and * $p < 0.10$.

potential responses. Latencies of the P100 component of the visually evoked potential response were significantly decreased on the first day of IFN treatment as well as after one week on therapy with IFN. Likewise, latencies of the major components of the auditory evoked brainstem potential response decreased during therapy with IFN, with this effect reaching significance for the Vn component. Shortened latencies of stimulus evoked potential components indicate an accelerated neural transmission in the afferent sensory paths of the brainstem and within the cortex after IFN.

Although patients developing high fever after IFN were not tested, a moderate increase in body temperature averaging 1.0 °C reached significance during therapy with IFN-γ (Table 1). Therefore, in the case of IFN-γ part of the increase in brain excitability as indicated by EEG and evoked potential measures, may reflect non-specific consequences of enhanced body temperature. However, this increase in body temperature appeared to be too small to completely account for all the changes in brain electrophysiological measures. Also, patients treated with IFN-α displayed changes in EEG-activity and evoked potentials comparable with those treated with IFN-γ, although after IFN-α an increase in body temperature was lacking. Hence, apart from changes in body temperature, other factors such as hormonal changes must be taken into account as potential mediators of the central nervous effects of IFNs (Späth-Schwalbe et al., 1989). Yet, blood-borne IFN has also direct access to the brain (Habif et al., 1975; Brightman et al., 1975; Smith et al., 1985).

While the signs of increased brain excitability in patients treated with IFN-γ and IFN-α fit with a similar effect of IFN observed in neurons in culture (Calvet and Gresser, 1979), in another clinical trial (Mattson et al., 1983, 1987), therapy with IFN-α was found to increase latencies of visual and auditory evoked potentials and to slow EEG activity. IFN-γ, in that study had no effects on EEG and evoked potentials. One reason for this discrepancy may be that those experimentors evaluated the EEG and evoked potentials after extended epochs of IFN treatment while the present authors' experiments focussed on a rather limited period of 1 week of IFN treatment. Furthermore, recordings were obtained always within a few hours after the last IFN administration suggesting that the signs of increased brain excitability reflect primarily acute influences of the cytokine.

The effects of treatment with IFNs described here, appear to be also at variance with results from animals indicating a sleep enhancing effect of these cytokines. In particular, slow wave sleep (SWS) has been shown to be augmented after intraventricular and intravenous administration of IFN-α (Krüger et al., 1987). Such sleep inducing effects would be expected to increase power within the lower EEG frequency bands. Yet, no such changes could be demonstrated in our patients although some of them reported on feelings of fatigue and exhaustion. This pattern obviously parallels findings in monkeys who showed increased behavioral deactivation and signs of fatigue after administration of IFN-α with no concomittant increases in EEG slow wave activity (Reite et al., 1987).

Nevertheless, despite of these parallel observations in monkeys and men, descrepant results appear to prevail when comparing results from animals and from studies in human patients evaluating central nervous effects of cytokines. Therefore, it is conceivable that effects of cytokines on sleep differ depending on the species investigated. However, in light of obvious inconsistencies also among clinical studies conducted in cancer patients the more critical question seems to be whether from studies in patients any solid conclusions can be drawn as to the role of cytokines for the regulation of central nervous EEG activity and sleep under normal physiological conditions, at all. The patients examined in those studies were all severely ill suffering from a great variety of diseases. Typically the cytokines were administered at a rather high dose and for a prolonged period of time. Moreover, the diseases in these patients commonly require additional medication of different types which may interfere with the effects of the cytokine. Together, these points cast serious doubt as to whether clinical studies on the central nervous effects of cytokines can answer any question beyond that of a possible neurotoxic side effect of the therapy.

Effects of interleukin-6 in healthy men

As experience with the administration of some selected cytokines in animals and in patients has substantially increased, it seems now legitimate to start studying central nervous effects of these cytokines in healthy humans. In such studies effects of cytokines can be evaluated for doses inducing plasma concentrations within the range normally observed during infections.

Here, we concentrate on a first of a series of studies initiated in our laboratory which aimed to assess the effects of IL-6 on central nervous sleep in healthy humans (Späth-Schwalbe et al., 1996). Effects of a single subcutaneous administration of IL-6 at a rather low dose ($0.5\ \mu g/kg$ body weight) were investigated which should mimick endogenous changes in plasma IL-6 concentrations observed normally following mild acute infection.

IL-6 is primarily produced by monocytes and macrophages. It has been shown to stimulate hemopoesis, i.e., the generation of neutrophils, monocytes, and platelets. Moreover, in vitro, IL-6 has been shown to stimulate the differentiation of T and B lymphocytes, the production of IL-2, and the expression of IL-2 receptors (Kishimoto, 1989; Le et al., 1988; Noma et al., 1987). Together with TNF-α and IL-1, IL-6 belongs to the major endogenous mediators of the acute phase response (Akira et al., 1990; Van Snick, 1990; Nijsten et al., 1987). This response describes a complex set of immediate reactions during the inflammatory process initiated upon infection or tissue damage, which may help the organism to cope with these challenges (Baumann and Gauldie, 1994). Manifestations of the acute phase response include fever, activation of the immune system, alterations in metabolism, changes in hepatic synthesis of plasma proteins and hormone secretion. Increased sleepiness is a common experience during infectious diseases. Hence, it was supposed that, in the context of the acute phase response and together with other cytokines, IL-6 would promote sleep thereby supporting the development of primary immune defence.

To assess effects of IL-6 on central nervous sleep, we conducted a double-blind cross-over study in 16 healthy men (aged between 22 and 30 yr). Subjects were screened by a medical history and evaluation of sleep habits, a physical examination, laboratory investigations and electrocardiogram to exclude acute and chronic disease. Recombi-

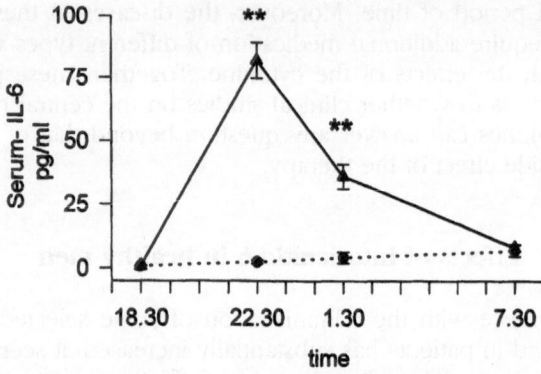

Fig. 1. Mean (±SEM) serum IL-6 concentrations after IL-6 administration (solid line) and placebo (dotted line). IL-6 (0.5 µg/kg body weight) or placebo were injected subcutaneously at 1900 h. $n = 16$. ** $p < 0.001$, for pairwise comparisons between the effects of IL-6 and placebo

nant human IL-6 (expressed in E. coli) versus placebo was injected at 1900 h prior to experimental nights. Lights were turned off at 2300 h to enable sleep. Subjects were awakened in the morning at 0700 h, and then stayed in bed (in a supine body position) until 0800 h. To determine various immunological and endocrinological parameters, blood was collected every 30 min between 1830 and 0800 h. During the wake periods prior to and after sleep blood pressure, heart rate and body temperature (sublingual) were measured every hour. At 2200 h and 0700 h in the morning, subjects were asked to complete an extensive checklist of adjectives (EWL) to assess feelings of activation, tiredness, and mood (Janke and Debus, 1978). In this list, a total of 161 adjectives are used to describe the subjects mood on 15 dimensions. For each adjective the man had to indicate whether or not it reflected his actual feelings.

Figure 1 shows the time course of IL-6 serum concentrations. After subcutaneous administration, peak concentrations of about 80 pg/ml were reached about 4 h later which, in fact, are comparable with those reached during mild acute infection. As expected, IL-6 also induced, with a delay of more than 6.5 h, a strong increase in serum concentrations of C-reactive protein. This influence is in line with the well documented effects of IL-6 on the synthesis of acute phase reactants (Weber et al., 1993; Gameren et al., 1994). However, contrasting with previous reports, IL-6 did not influence serum concentrations of IL-2, IFN-γ and IFN-α, and the expression of IL-2 receptors in T cells. There were also no changes in platelet counts after IL-6. An enhancing effect of IL-6 on the production of IL-2 and on the expression of IL-2 receptors was demonstrated in vitro (Kishimoto, 1989; Le et al., 1988; Noma et al., 1987). An increased expression of IL-2 receptors has been likewise revealed in patients after 21 days of daily injections of IL-6 at high doses of 30 μg/kg body weight (Weber et al., 1993). Also, platelet counts have been found to be increased in patients during prolonged IL-6 treatment with the effect emerging not until the third day of treatment (Weber et al., 1993; Gameren et al., 1994). Obviously, duration and dose of IL-6 treatment can account for the discrepant immunological influences of IL-6 reported in in-vitro-studies, in studies in patients and in healthy humans. Higher doses and prolonged treatment may be required to invoke effects in-vivo comparable with those observed in-vitro. Also, in-vivo a regulatory influence of IL-6 on other cytokines may not manifest itself in an enhanced release of these cytokines into the blood stream.

The single subcutaneous administration of IL-6 induced distinct changes of the nocturnal sleep architecture which are summarized in Fig. 2 and Table 2. Total sleep time and sleep onset were comparable in both the placebo and IL-6 conditions. IL-6 injection significantly increased the latency of REM sleep, and reduced the time as well as the per cent of time spent in REM sleep. Separate evaluation of the first and second half of nighttime revealed that the reduction in REM sleep was somewhat more consistent during the first ($p < 0.001$) than second half of the night ($p = 0.06$). IL-6 decreased time in SWS during the first half of the night, but the amount of SWS was twofold increased in the second half of the night ($p < 0.005$). Thus, for the entire night differences in time in SWS following IL-6 and placebo remained non-significant. Time spent in the other sleep stages and awake was not affected by IL-6.

The effects of IL-6 on sleep were accompanied by changes in mood, as determined by the adjective check list. These effect concentrated on measures taken at 2200 h prior to nocturnal sleep. Self reported mood measured in the morning after sleep yielded virtually identical scores following administration of placebo and IL-6. At 2200 h, i.e., 3 hours after administration of IL-6 subjects felt less concentrated and more tired and deactivated than following placebo. Also, IL-6 substantially lowered scores on the "high spirits" dimension of the mood adjective checklist (Fig. 3).

Part of the changes in sleep and mood observed after IL-6 may reflect effects secondary to actions of the cytokine on body temperature and endocrine secretion. After IL-6 injection, body temperature gradually increased on average by 0.8 °C, compared with placebo at 2300 h ($p < 0.001$). Body temperature was still slightly but significantly enhanced at the time of awakening at 0800 h. Substantial increases in body temperature have been found to be accompanied by increases in SWS and reduced REM sleep in previous experiments (Horne and Moore, 1985; Horne and Reid, 1985; Bunnell and Horvath, 1985). However, in a recent study (Cajochen et al., 1992) slight elevations of body temperature – comparable with those observed here after IL-6 – were not linked to substantial changes in SWS. Moreover, in contrast with elevations of body temperature, IL-6 during the first half of sleep time significantly

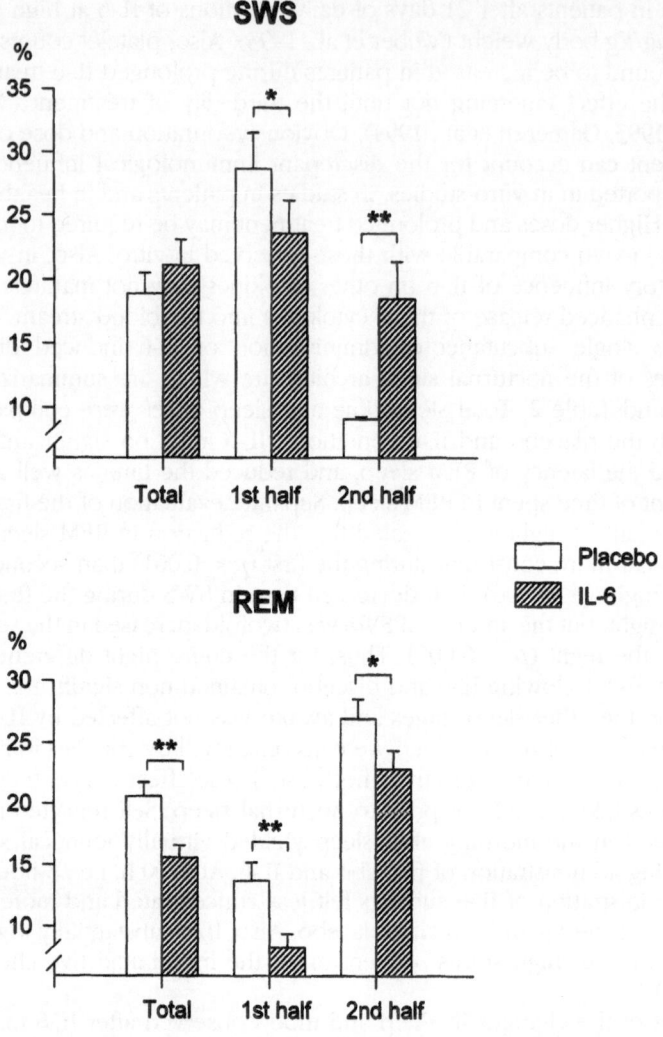

Fig. 2. Mean (±SEM) per cent of time spent in slow wave sleep (SWS; top) and rapid eye movement sleep (REM; bottom) for the total sleep period, first and second half of sleep after IL-6 (0.5 µg/kg body weight; hatched bars) and placebo (empty bars). * $P < 0.05$; ** $P < 0.01$ for pairwise comparisons between the effects of IL-6 and placebo

decreased the time spent in SWS. Thus, the increase in body temperature may have contributed to the decreased time in REM sleep after IL-6, but would not explain that the cytokine shifted the major epochs of SWS from the first half into the second half of the night.

time: 22.00 h

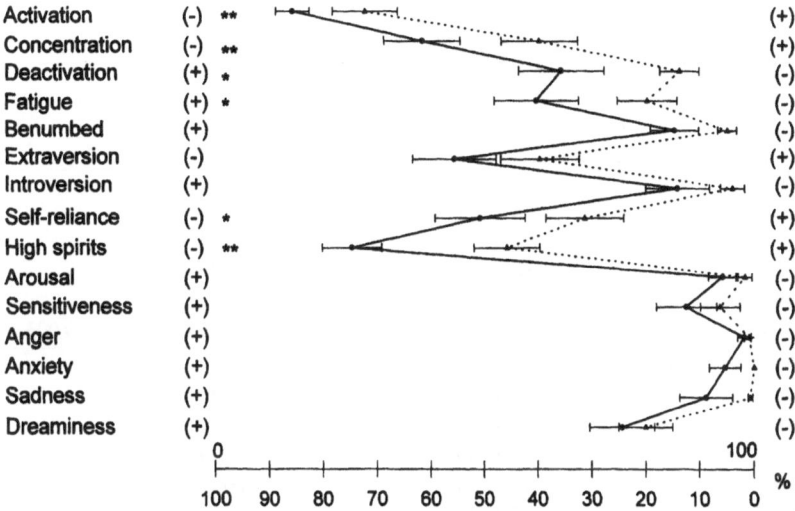

Activation	(-) **		(+)
Concentration	(-) **		(+)
Deactivation	(+) *		(-)
Fatigue	(+) *		(-)
Benumbed	(+)		(-)
Extraversion	(-)		(+)
Introversion	(+)		(-)
Self-reliance	(-) *		(+)
High spirits	(-) **		(+)
Arousal	(+)		(-)
Sensitiveness	(+)		(-)
Anger	(+)		(-)
Anxiety	(+)		(-)
Sadness	(+)		(-)
Dreaminess	(+)		(-)

Fig. 3. Profiles of mood as measured by an extended adjective checklist (EWL, Janke and Debus, 1978) 3 hours after injection of IL-6 (0.5 µg/kg body weight) and placebo (administered at 1900 h). IL-6, solid lines; placebo, dotted lines. * $P < 0.05$; ** $P < 0.01$ for pairwise comparisons between the effects of IL-6 and placebo

With regard to endocrine activity, IL-6 exerted most pronounced effects on the secretion of thyroid stimulating hormone (TSH) and on pituitary adrenal secretory activity (Fig. 4). Plasma growth hormone concentrations were not affected by IL-6. Plasma TSH levels were similar before drug administration (1900 h) on both nights. On the placebo nights, the typical nocturnal TSH surge, beginning before sleep onset, was observed. TSH concentrations remained increased during the first hours of sleep and then declined to reach a minimum during the early morning hours. IL-6 almost completely blunted the nocturnal TSH surge, and kept TSH levels substantially decreased throughout the night. The decrease proved to be significant between 2300 and 0600 h in the morning.

While plasma TSH concentrations were decreased after IL-6, the cytokine exerted a marked stimulatory effect on the release of adrenocorticotropin (ACTH) and cortisol (Fig. 4). While on placebo nights, ACTH/cortisol plasma concentrations reached the typical diurnal nadir during the early evening and the first hours of sleep, following IL-6 pituitary-adrenal secretory activity remained at an enhanced level throughout the night. Compared with the effects of placebo, the increase in ACTH/cortisol plasma concentrations following IL-6 reached significance within one hour after subcutaneous administration of the

112   J. Born and E. Späth-Schwalbe

Table 2. Total sleep time, sleep onset, absolute and per cent of sleep time spent in each sleep stage after placebo and IL-6

Parameter	Placebo (mean ± SEM)	IL-6 (mean ± SEM)	P-value <
Time (min)			
Sleep onset latency	20.3 (4.7)	16.4 (2.8)	
Sleep time	445.0 (5.3)	448.9 (3.3)	
Per cent			
W	3.8 (0.9)	4.2 (0.6)	
S1	9.9 (1.8)	9.3 (1.4)	
S2	47.0 (1.8)	49.9 (2.1)	
SWS	18.9 (1.6)	21.1 (2.0)	
REM	20.6 (1.1)	15.6 (1.0)	0.003
Per cent, 1st half			
W	3.5 (1.6)	3.8 (0.7)	
S1	8.8 (2.2)	13.3 (2.3)	
S2	45.3 (2.7)	51.1 (2.8)	
SWS	28.7 (2.8)	23.6 (2.6)	0.05
REM	13.7 (1.5)	8.3 (1.1)	0.001
Per cent, 2nd half			
W	4.2 (1.0)	4.6 (1.1)	
S1	11.0 (2.0)	5.2 (1.5)	0.002
S2	48.7 (1.8)	48.8 (1.9)	
SWS	9.1 (0.2)	18.5 (2.9)	0.005
REM	26.9 (1.6)	22.8 (1.5)	0.06
Latency (min, with reference to sleep onset)			
S2	6.9 (1.0)	8.4 (1.0)	0.06
SWS	19.9 (1.3)	31.3 (9.1)	
REM	92.0 (9.6)	128.4 (16.1)	0.002

W wake; *S1, S2* sleep stage 1 and 2; *SWS* slow wave sleep, i.e., sleep stages 3 + 4; *REM* rapid eye movement sleep. Significant *p*-values determined from multivariate analysis of variance; degrees of freedom; 1.15

cytokine. ACTH and cortisol levels remained significantly enhanced after IL-6 throughout the first half of the night until 0130 and 0230 h, respectively. During the rest of the night, cortisol concentrations did not differ substantially between the placebo and IL-6 conditions. But, ACTH concentrations during the late night appeared to be somewhat lower following IL-6 than placebo. Considering that glucocorticoids have been demonstrated to suppress pulsatile TSH secretion for several hours, the pronounced increase in cortisol concentrations after IL-6 may at least partly explain the inhibitory effect of the cytokine on TSH secretion (Wilber and Utiger, 1969; Re et al., 1976; Brabant et al., 1987).

The effects of IL-6 on sleep probably cannot be reduced to its sup-

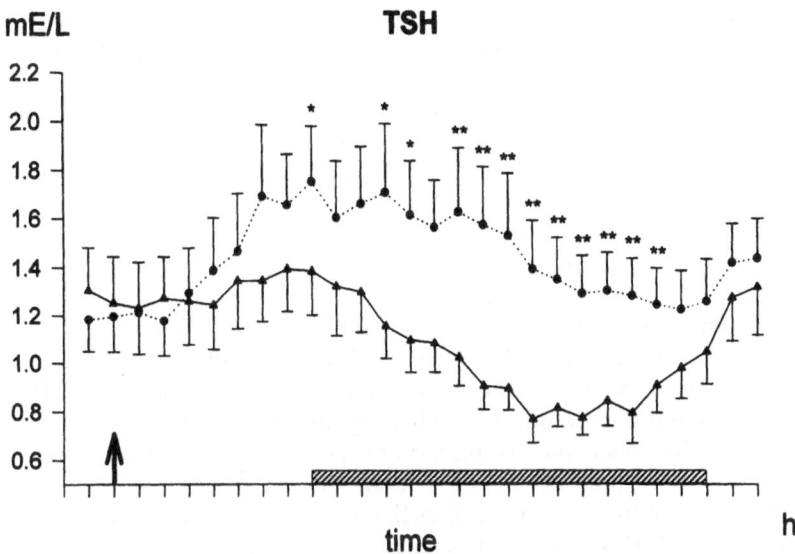

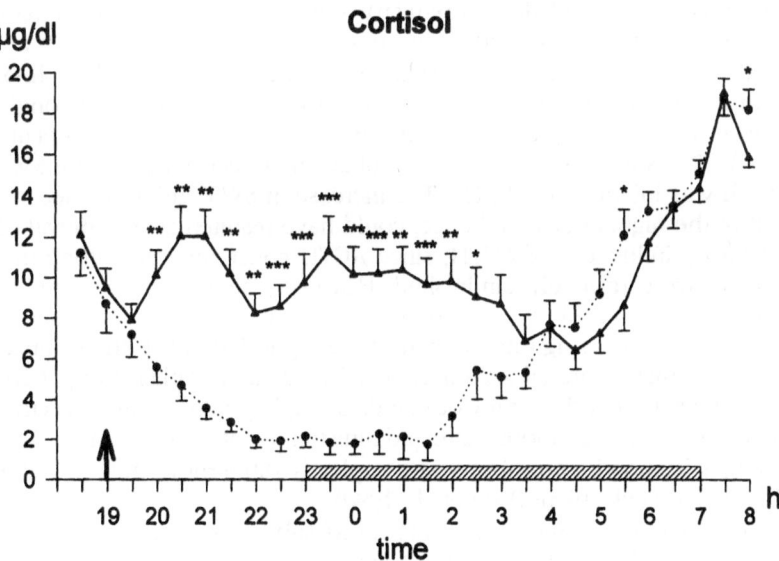

Fig. 4. Mean (±SEM) nocturnal profiles of plasma TSH (top) and cortisol (bottom) after placebo (dotted lines, filled circles) and IL-6 (0.5 μg/kg bwt; solid lines, filled triangles) administration at 1900 h (arrow). Horizontal bar (hatched) indicates sleep period. * $P < 0.05$; ** $P < 0.01$; *** $P < 0.001$ for pairwise comparisons between the effects of IL-6 and placebo

pressing influence on TSH release. Studies in hypothyroid patients and in healthy humans after administration of thyrotropin releasing hormone (TRH) yielded inconclusive results which did support the view that low plasma levels of TSH could result in sleep changes similar to those observed after IL-6 (Alford et al., 1973; Kales et al., 1967; Nakazawa et al., 1979). It should be considered also that the suppression of TSH levels may have contributed to the impaired mood after IL-6. In some depressed patients, TSH responses to TRH have been found to be reduced (Whybrow and Prange, 1981). Moreover, administration of synthetic TRH has been reported to produce a transient antidepressive effect, although findings overall remained controversial (Whybrow and Prange, 1981; Prange et al., 1979). However, regardless of whether or not TSH improves mood, it is to emphasize that the suppression of TSH after IL-6 in our experiments reached significance not until 2300 h (i.e., 4 hours after subcutaneous injection of IL-6) while the striking changes in mood were present already 3 hours after IL-6 injection. Thus, the early onset of mood changes after IL-6 makes an essential contribution of reduced TSH release to these changes very unlikely.

With respect to the effects of IL-6 on sleep, a mediating role of pituitary-adrenal secretory activity has to be considered. The finding of a stimulating effect of IL-6 on pituitary-adrenal secretory activity agrees with several foregoing studies in animals and patients (Naitoh et al., 1988; Mastorakos et al., 1993; Späth-Schwalbe et al., 1994). Like IL-6, both administration of ACTH and cortisol has been found to strongly reduce time spent in REM sleep in a previous experiment (Born et al., 1989). That study also indicated an enhancing effect of cortisol on SWS which was inhibited by ACTH. The increase in SWS during the second half of the night after IL-6, hence, could have resulted from removal of inhibitory influences of ACTH, since ACTH concentrations during this interval were relatively diminished. However, neither the changes in cortisol nor in ACTH concentrations can explain the reducing influence of IL-6 on SWS during the first part of the night. Moreover, the stimulation of pituitary-adrenal secretion after IL-6 cannot explain the pattern of changes in mood. In previous studies employing the same adjective check list to assess mood, after administration of cortisol and ACTH changes in mood were observed completely different from those after IL-6 (Plihal et al., 1996; Born et al., 1990).

The changes of mood, i.e., increased subjective tiredness and deactivation and low scores on the "high spirits" scale, after IL-6 closely resembled the feelings often reported during infections. The findings lend themselves to propose that cytokines released upon infectious challenge are the essential factors causing the typical sickness-related changes in mood. Interestingly, these feelings included increased tiredness and fatigue although subsequent sleep recordings did not indicate enhanced but reduced SWS during early sleep. A similar pattern of increased subjective tiredness without concommittant slowing of the EEG activity has been observed in patients treated with IFNs (see above) and also in monkeys after administration of IFN-α (Reite et al., 1987). Taken together, these results suggest that upon infection IL-6, in concert with other cytokines, exerts an acute inhibitory effect on the expression of orthodoxical sleep (i.e., SWS) although propensity for sleep is increasing.

In conclusion, the data suggest that IL-6 released during infection, inflammation or trauma, substantially alters mood and sleep architecture. IL-6 induced mood changes reminiscent of a feeling of sickness and increased subjective fatigue. However, simultaneously SWS was delayed and the time in REM sleep was distinctly suppressed after IL-6. While the suppression of REM sleep and the increase in SWS during late sleep may in part be mediated by the IL-6 induced stimulation of pituitary-adrenal secretory activity, the acute suppression of SWS as well as the impaired mood after IL-6 involves other mechanisms. IL-6 also decreased plasma concentrations of TSH and increased body temperature. However, considering the late onset of the decrease in TSH and effects of TSH and body temperature reported in other studies, these factors cannot be taken to explain the acute impairing effects of IL-6 on SWS and mood. Thus, it remains possible that these changes reflect a more direct effect of the cytokine on brain function.

The central nervous changes after IL-6 may be regarded as manifestations of the acute phase response mediated by this and several other cytokines. To what extent these changes serve to support the organism's coping with an infectious challenge remains to be elucidated. Together, neither evaluation of effects of IFN in patients nor evaluation of effects of IL-6 in healthy subjects provided any evidence for a sleep promoting effect of proinflammatory cytokines in humans. This finding contrasts with results from animal studies that have indicated somnogenic influences of IFNs whereas IL-6 in rats left sleep unaffected (Krüger et al., 1987; Opp et al., 1989). These obvious discrepancies underline the importance of experiments in humans to determine the role of cytokines in the regulation of sleep and brain activity under normal physiological conditions in this species. Considering findings of increased levels of proinflammatory cytokines in subgroups of psychiatric patients (e.g., Appelberg et al., 1997; Ganguli et al., 1993), the activated release of such cytokines could be one factor among others contributing to the severe sleep disturbances in these patients.

Acknowledgements

This work was supported by the Volkswagen-Stiftung (E. S. S.) and the Deutsche Forschungsgemeinschaft (J. B.). We thank A. Otterbein for helpful assistance with preparing the manuscript.

116   J. Born and E. Späth-Schwalbe

References

Akira S, Hirano T, Taga T, Kishimoto T (1990) Biology of multifunctional cytokines: IL 6 and related molecules (IL 1 and TNF). FASEB J 4:2860–2867

Alford FP, Baker HW, Burger HG, de Kretser DM, Hudson B, Johns MW, Masterson JP (1973) Temporal patterns of integrated plasma hormone levels during sleep and wakefulness. J Clin Endocrinol Metab 37:841–847

Appelberg B, Katila H, Rimon R (1997) Plasma interleukin-1β and sleep architecture in schizophrenia and other non-affective psychoses. Psychosom Med 59:529–532

Baumann H, Gauldie J (1994) The acute phase response. Immunol Today 15:74–80

Born J, Späth-Schwalbe E, Pietrowsky R, Porzsolt F, Fehm HL (1989) Neurophysiological effects of recombinant interferon-gamma and alpha in man. Clin Physiol Biochem 7:119–127

Born J, Späth-Schwalbe E, Schwakenhofer H, Kern W, Fehm HL (1989) Influences of corticotropin-releasing hormone, adrenocorticotropin, and cortisol on sleep in normal man. J Clin Endocrinol Metab 68:904–911

Born J, Bathelt B, Pietrowsky R, Pauschinger P, Fehm HL (1990) Influences of peripheral adrenocorticotropin 1-39 (ACTH) and human corticotropin releasing hormone (h-CRH) on human auditory evoked potentials (AEP). Psychopharmacol 101:34–38

Born J, Lange T, Hansen K, Mölle M, Fehm HL (1997) Effects of sleep and circadian rhythm on human circulating immune cells. J Immunol 158:4454–4464

Brabant G, Brabant A, Ranft U, Ocran K, Köhrle J, Hesch RD, von zur Mühlen A (1987) Circadian and pulsatile thyrotropin secretion in euthyroid man under the influence of thyroid hormone and glucocorticoid administration. J Clin Endocrinol Metab 65:83–88

Brightman MW, Prescott L, Reese TS (1975) Intercellular junctions of special ependyma. In: Knigge S, Scott WT, Kobayashi Y, Ishii Y (eds) Brain endocrine interaction. Karger, Basel, pp 146–165

Bunnell DE, Horvath SM (1985) Effects of body heating during sleep interruption. Sleep 8:274–282

Cajochen C, Dijk DJ, Borbély AA (1992) Dynamics of EEG slow wave activity and core body temperature in human sleep after exposure to bright light. Sleep 15:337–343

Calvet M, Gresser I (1979) Interferon enhances the excitability of cultured neurons. Nature 278:558–560

Dinges DF, Douglas SD, Zaugg L, Campbell DE, McMann JM, Whitehouse WG, Orne EC, Kapoor SC, Icaza E, Orne MT (1994) Leukocytosis and natural killer cell function parallel neurobehavioral fatigue induced by 64 hours of sleep deprivation. J Clin Invest 93:1930–1939

Gameren MM, Willemse PHB, Mulder NH, Limburg PC, Groen HJM, Vellenga E, de Vries EGE (1994) Effects of recombinant human interleukin-6 in cancer patients: a phase I–II study. Blood 84:1434–1441

Ganguli R, Brar JS, Chengappa KN, Yang ZW, Nimgaonkar VL, Rabin BS (1993) Autoimmunity in schizophrenia: a review of recent findings. Ann Med 25:489–496

Habif DV, Lipton R, Cantell K (1975) Interferon crosses blood-cerebrospinal fluid barrier in monkeys. Proc Soc Exp Biol Med 149:287–289

Hirano T, Akira S, Taga T, Kishimoto T (1990) Biological and clinical aspects of interleukin 6. Immunol Today 11:443–449

Horne JA, Moore VJ (1985) Sleep effects of exercise with and without additional body cooling. Electroencephalogr Clin Neurophysiol 60:33–38

Horne JA, Reid AJ (1985) Night-time sleep EEG changes following body heating in a warm bath. Electroencephalogr Clin Neurophysiol 60:154–157

Janke W, Debus G (1978) Die Eigenschaftswörterliste EWL. Eine mehrdimensionale Methode zur Beschreibung von Aspekten des Befindens. Hogrefe, Göttingen

Kales A, Heuser G, Jacobson A, Kales JD, Hanley J, Zweizig JR, Paulson MJ (1967) All night sleep studies in hypothyroid patients, before and after treatment. J Clin Endocrinol Metab 27:1593–1599

Kishimoto T (1989) The biology of interleukin-6. Blood 74:1–10

Krüger JM, Karnovsky ML (1995) Sleep as a neuroimmune phenomenon: a brief historical perspective. Adv Neuroimmunol 5:5–12

Krüger JM, Walter J, Dianrello CA, Wolff SM, Chedid L (1984) Sleep-promoting effects of endogenous pyrogen. Am J Physiol 246:R994–999

Krüger JM, Dinarello CA, Shoham S, Davenne D, Walter J, Kubillus S (1987) Interferon alpha-2 enhances slow-wave sleep in rabbits. Int J Immunopharmacol 9: 23–30

Krüger JM, Obal F, Opp L, Toth L, Johannsen L, Cady AB (1990) Somnogenic cytokines and models concerning their effects on sleep. Yale J Biol Med 106:97–100

Le JM, Fredrickson G, Reis LFL, Diamantsein T, Hirano T, Kishimoto T, Vilcek J (1988) Interleukin 2-dependent and interleukin 2-independent pathways of regulation of thymocyte function by interleukin-6. Proc Natl Acad Sci USA 85:8643–8647

Mastorakos G, Chrousos GP, Weber JS (1993) Recombinant interleukin-6 activates the hypothalamic-pituitary-adrenal axis in humans. J Clin Endocrinol Metab 77: 1690–1694

Mattson K, Niiranen A, Iivanainen M, Färkkila M, Bergström L, Holsti LR, Kauppinen HL, Cantell K (1983) Neurotoxicity of interferon. Cancer Treat Rep 67:958–961

Mattson K, Holsti LR, Niiranen A, Pyrhönen S, Färkkilä M, Härtel G, Standertskiölt-Nordenstam CG, Cantell K (1987) Comparison of clinical toxicity of natural alpha and recombinant gamma interferon. In: Cantell ST, Schellekens V (eds) The biology of interferon system 1986. Nijhoff, Dordrecht

Naitoh Y, Fukata J, Tominaga T, Nakai T, Tamai S, Mori K, Imura H (1988) Interleukin-6 stimulates the secretion of adrenocorticotropic hormone in conscious, freely-moving rats. Biochem Biophys Res Commun 155:1459–1463

Nakazawa Y, Kotorii T, Horikawa S, Kororii M, Ohshima M, Hasuzawa H (1979) Individual variations in the effects of flurazepam, clorazepate, L-dopa and thyrotropin-releasing hormone on REM sleep in man. Psychopharmacology 60: 203–206

Nijsten MWN, De Groot ER, Ten Duis HJ, Klasen HJ, Hack CE, Aarden LA (1987) Serum levels of interleukin-6 and acute phase responses. Lancet ii:921

Noma T, Mizuta T, Rosen A, Hirano T, Kishimoto T, Honjo T (1987) Enhancement of the interleukin 2 receptr expression on T cells by multiple B-lymphotopic lymphokines. Immunol Lett 15:249–253

Opp M, Obal F Jr, Cady AB, Johannsen L, Krüger JM (1989) Interleukin-6 is pyrogenic but not somnogenic. Physiol Behav 45:1069–1072

118   J. Born and E. Späth-Schwalbe

Plihal W, Krug R, Pietrowsky R, Fehm HL, Born J (1996) Corticosteroid receptor mediated effects on mood in humans. Psychoneuroendocrinology 21:513–523

Prange AJ, Loosen PT, Neuroff CB (1979) Peptides: application to research in nervous and mental disorders. In: Fielding S (ed) New frontier of psychotropic drug research. Futura, New York

Reite M, Laudenslager M, Jones J, Crnic L, Kaemingk K (1987) Interferon decreases REM latency. Biol Psychiatry 22:104–107

Shoham S, Davenne D, Cady AB, Dinarello CA, Krüger JM (1987) Recombinant tumor necrosis factor and interleukin-1 enhance slow-wave sleep in rabbits. Am J Physiol 253:R142–149

Smith RA, Norris F, Palmer D, Bernhardt L, Wills RJ (1985) Distribution of alpha interferon in serum and cerebrospinal fluid after systemic administration. Clin Pharmacol Ther 37:85–88

Späth-Schwalbe E, Porzsolt F, Kigel W, Born J, Kloss B, Fehm HL (1989) Elevated plasma cortisol levels during interferon-γ treatment. Immunopharmacology 17: 141–145

Späth-Schwalbe E, Born J, Schrezenmeier H, Bornstein SR, Stromeyer P, Drechsler S, Fehm HL, Porzsolt F (1994) Interleukin-6 stimulates the hypothalamus-pituitary-adrenocortical axis in man. J Clin Endocrinol Metab 79:1212–1214

Späth-Schwalbe E, Hansen K, Schmidt F, Bornstein S, Burger K, Fehm HL, Born J (1996) Effects of recombinant interleukin-6 in healthy men. A: Analysis of nocturnal hormone secretion and sleep after interleukin-6 administration (submitted)

Toth LA (1995) Sleep, sleep deprivation and infectious disease: studies in animals. Adv Neuroimmunol 5:79–92

Van Snick J (1990) Interleukin-6: an overview. Annu Rev Immunol 8:253–278

Weber J, Yang JC, Topalian SL, Parkinson DR, Schwartentruber DS, Ettinghausen SE, Gunn H, Mixon A, Kim H, Cole D (1993) Phase I trial of subcutaneous interleukin-6 in patients with advanced malignancies. J Clin Oncol 11:499–506

Whybrow RP, Prange AJ (1981) A hypothesis of thyroid-catecholamine-receptor interaction. Arch Gen Psychiatry 38:106–113

Wilber JF, Utiger RD (1969) The effect of glucocorticoids on thyrotropin secretion. J Clin Invest 48:2096–2103

Correspondence: Prof. Dr. J. Born, Klinische Forschergruppe – Klinische Neuro-endokrinologie, Medizinische Universität Lübeck, Ratzeburger Allee 160, Haus 23a, D-23538 Lübeck, Federal Republic of Germany.

Role of cingulate gyrus during Wisconsin card sorting test: a single photon emission computed tomography (SPECT) study

A. M. Catafau[1], E. Parellada[2], F. Lomeña[1], and M. Bernardo[2]

[1] Grup Investigador en Psiquiatria, Fundació Clínic, and
[2] Nuclear Medicine and Psychiatry Departments, Hospital Clínic,
Universitat de Barcelona, Barcelona, Spain

Background

Single Photon Emission Computed Tomography, commonly known as SPECT, is a functional neuroimaging technique which provides information on cerebral perfusion. Perfusion SPECT images reflect neuronal activity, due to the relationship between cerebral blood flow and metabolism. Thus, brain SPECT can be used for the study of the normal brain, but since symptoms are a reflection of brain activity, this technique can also be helpful in studies of brain pathology, providing some insight into the pathophysiology of schizophrenia, for example.

Using SPECT, the normal or pathological brain can be evaluated both under baseline conditions (or "at rest") and under activation, which includes motor, sensory, pharmacologic or cognitive processes. Cognitive processes are of great interest, because they cannot be studied in animals. Frontal cognitive tests, such as the Wisconsin Card Sorting Test (WCST), have been the most widely used in schizophrenia research, since the prefrontal cortex has been found to be dysfunctional in this disorder (Berman and Weinberger, 1991; Andreasen et al., 1994). However, functional neuroimaging results in this area are inconsistent, due to differences in the selection criteria for study populations and in the methodology applied (Andreasen et al., 1992). For example, using SPECT, the rCBF estimation is based on the uptake of tracer found in selected "regions of interest" (ROIs), which can be drawn in many different ways depending on the purpose of the study (George et al., 1991). These ROIs can also be more or less detailed depending on the spatial resolution of the system used.

In a previous SPECT study of 25 unmedicated schizophrenic patients and 15 age and sex matched normal subjects, we reported that during the WCST performance, the control group showed a significant rCBF increase in all prefrontal regions studied, while no rCBF increase was found in the same areas in the schizophrenic group, especially in the left hemisphere (Catafau et al., 1994a; Bernardo et al., 1996). However, there was not the same degree of change in all the frontal regions. A greater rCBF increase in the cingulate region than in the dorso-lateral prefrontal cortex was found. This fact encouraged us to study the cingulate region independently.

The cingulate gyri are paired cortical structures located in the midsagital plane of the brain, superiorly surrounding the corpus callosum. The cingulate gyrus is classically divided into a large anterior part, corresponding to the frontal lobe, and a smaller posterior part. It is extensively connected with other limbic structures, as well as with the thalamus and the associative cortex (temporal, parietal, frontal) (Isaacson, 1982). Although functions of the cingulate gyrus are not fully known, the anterior part has been classically implied in expression and modulation of emotion, memory processing, exploratory behavior, maternal behavior and attention to visual stimulus (Isaacson, 1982; McLean, 1990). More recently, PET studies have shown the cingulate to be implicated in attentional mechanisms (Petersen et al., 1988; Pardo et al., 1990; Dolan et al., 1995). Attentional mechanisms are implied in the pathophysiology of important psychiatric disorders, such as schizophrenia (Andreasen et al., 1994) and mood disorders (Bench et al., 1992). In addition, attention is a function required for the performance of frontal cognitive tests used in the neuropsychological evaluation of these disorders. However, the cingulate gyrus is not always considered independent of the prefrontal cortex in SPECT studies of frontal cognitive activation, as was the case in our previous works (Parellada et al., 1994; Catafau et al., 1994b), in which both structures were included in the same region of interest, yet the most striking changes during WCST activation were visually located in the cingulate region. In addition, Dolan et al. (1995), using PET and a verbal fluency test have recently demonstrated a selective activation of the anterior cingulate cortex in normal subjects, as well as a selective activation failure in this structure in unmedicated schizophrenic patients, which is significantly enhanced after dopaminergic manipulation with apomorphine.

Now, with the new generation gammacameras, the spatial resolution of the brain SPECT images has improved, allowing one to draw more precise ROIs, and thus to separate the cingulate from the remaining frontal cortex for an independent evaluation of each structure.

Furthermore, in resting-activation SPECT studies, rCBF changes due to order effects should be considered, since higher rCBF at first measurement than at second or subsequent measurements has been reported as an adaptation to the test conditions using the 133-Xe technique (Risberg et al., 1977; Warach et al., 1987).

Thus, the aims of the present study were:

1. To investigate the effect of the Wisconsin Card Sorting Test (WCST) in normal subjects on frontal rCBF, independently evaluating the cingulate from the remaining frontal cortex.

2. To study the effect of order on the rCBF changes by randomizing the order of resting and activated HMPAO-SPECTs.

Method

Two ^{99m}Tc-HMPAO SPECTs (at rest and during WCST performance) were performed in a randomized order 48 hours apart on 13 right-handed normal volunteers (9 male, 4 female, mean age 19.8 ± 0.8 yrs.). Brain SPECTs were carried out on a double-headed system (Elscint-Helix HR), fitted with two fanbeam collimators (FWHM 9 mm in the transaxial plane). After 3-D software realignment (Pavía et al., 1994), region/cerebellar ratios were obtained using a template of ROIs placed in all cases by the same investigator, as desribed elsewere (Catafau et al., 1996). The regions studied were: The anterior frontal region representing the prefrontal area, the posterior frontal region including the motor area, and the anterior and posterior regions of the frontal aspect of the cingulate gyrus. An activation score, resulting from subtracting resting from activated ratios, was also obtained for each region. For statistics, the Wilcoxon test (rest–activation comparisons), and the Mann–Whitney U-test (order comparisons) were used.

Results and conclusions

Our results showed that the left anterior cingulate as well as the left posterior frontal regions showed a significant rCBF increase during the WCST ($p < 0.033$). No significant differences were found in the remaining frontal regions, although 9 out of the 13 subjects studied showed an rCBF increase in the left and right prefrontal regions and right anterior cingulate as well.

Referring to order comparisons, no differences were found either in the activation scores or in the WCST scores between subjects having the resting SPECT first and subjects having the resting SPECT last.

These results suggest that the WCST predominantly activates the left anterior cingulate cortex, a limbic region that has been implicated in the attentional mechanisms involved in this test. Furthermore, the motor task implied in the act of matching cards during the WCST could explain the activation of the left posterior frontal region. In addition, no order effect was found in this study.

These findings illustrate the advantage of independently evaluating the cingulate gyrus and the prefrontal cortex in SPECT studies of cognitive tests used to assess frontal function. This may be particularly appropriate when studying psychiatric disorders such as schizophrenia and mood disorders, in which the cingulate gyrus could play a relevant role.

References

Andreasen NC, Rezai K, Alliger R, Swayze II VW, Flaum M, Kirchner P, Cohen G, O'Leary DS (1992) Hypofrontality in neuroleptic-naïve patients and in patients with chronic schizophrenia: assessment with xenon 133 single-photon emission computed tomography and the Tower of London. Arch Gen Psychiatry 49:943–958

Andreasen NC, Swayze VW, Flaum M, O'Leary DS, Alliger R (1994) The neural mechanisms of mental phenomena. In: Andreasen NC (ed) Schizophrenia. From mind to molecule. American Psychiatric Press, Washington, pp 49–91

Bench CJ, Friston KJ, Braun RG, Scott LC, Frackowiac RSJ, Dolan RJ (1992) The anatomy of melancholia-focal abnormalities of cerebral blood flow in major depression. Psychol Med 22:607–615

Berman KF, Weinberger DR (1991) Functional localization in the brain in schizophrenia. In: Annual review of psychiatry: schizophrenia. American Psychiatric Press, Washington, pp 24–59

Bernardo M, Parellada E, Catafau AM, Lomeña F (1996) SPECT imaging in schizophrenic patients. Partnerships 1996 Annual Meeting Syllabus and Proceedings Summary. America's mental health. American Psychiatric Association Annual Meeting, New York, May 4–9, pp 103–104

Catafau AM, Parellada E, Huguet M, Lomeña F, Bernardo M, Pavía J, Ros D, Setoain J (1994a) HMPAO brain SPECT in unmedicated acute schizophrenic patients: relationship with psychopathology and frontal cognitive activation. Eur J Nucl Med 21:S80

Catafau AM, Parellada E, Lomeña F, Bernardo M, Pavía J, Ros D, Setoain J, González-Monclús E (1994b) Prefrontal and temporal blood flow in schizophrenia: resting and activation technetium-99m-HMPAO SPECT patterns in young neuroleptic-naive patients with acute disease. J Nucl Med 35:935–941

Catafau AM, Lomeña FJ, Pavia J, Parellada E, Bernardo M, Setoain J, Tolosa E (1996) Regional cerebral blood flow pattern in normal young and aged volunteers. A ^{99m}Tc-HMPAO SPECT study. Eur J Nucl Med 23:1329–1337

Dolan RJ, Fletcher P, Frith CD, Friston KJ, Frackowiack RSJ, Grasby PM (1995) Dopaminergic modulation of impaired cognitive activation in the anterior cingulate cortex in schizophrenia. Nature 378:180–182

George MS, Ring HA, Costa DC, Ell PJ, Kouris K, Jarrit PH (eds) (1991) Neuroactivation and neuroimaging with SPECT. Springer, London

Isaacson RL (1982) The limbic system. Plenum Press, New York, pp 99–108

McLean PD (1990) An anatomical framework for considering limbic functions. In: The triune brain in evolution. Plenum Press, New York, pp 269–313

Pardo JV, Pardo PJ, Janer KW, Raichle ME (1990) The anterior cingulate cortex mediates processing selection in the Stroop attentional conflict paradigm. Proc Natl Acad Sci 87:256–259

Parellada E, Catafau AM, Bernardo M, Lomeña F, Gonzalez-Monclús F, Setoain J (1994) Prefrontal dysfunction in young acute neuroleptic-naive schizophrenic patients: a resting and activation SPECT study. Psychiatry Res Neuroimaging 55: 131–139

Pavía J, Ros D, Catafau AM, Lomeña F, Huguet M, Setoain J (1994) 3-D realignment of activation brain SPECT studies. Eur J Nucl Med 21:1298–1302

Petersen SE, Fox PT, Posner MI, Minntun M, Raichle ME (1988) Positron emission tomographic studies of the cortical anatomy of single-word processing. Nature 331:585–589

Risberg J, Maximillian VA, Prohovnik I (1977) Changes of cortical activity patterns during habituation to a reasoning test: a study with the 133-Xe technique for measuring regional cerebral blood flow. Neuropsychologia 15:793–798

Warach S, Gur RC, Gur RE, Skolnick B, Obrist W, Reivich M (1987) The reproducibility of the 133-Xe inhalation method technique in resting studies: task order and sex-related effects in healthy young adults. J Cereb Blood Flow Metab 7:702–708

Correspondence: Dr. A. M. Catafau, Servicio de Medicina Nuclear, Hospital de Sant Pau, San Antonio M. Claret 167, E-08025 Barcelona, Spain.

SpringerNeurology

Y. Mizuno, M. B. H. Youdim, D. B. Calne, R. Horowski,
W. Poewe, P. Riederer (eds.)

Advances in Research on Neurodegeneration
Volume 3 & 4

1997. 46 figures. VIII, 280 pages.
Cloth DM 215,–, öS 1505,–
ISBN 3-211-82935-0
Special edition of "Journal of Neural Transmission, Suppl. 49, 1997"

The "International Winter Conferences on Neurodegeneration" have become an established forum to discuss various aspects of basic and clinical topics related to the underlying mechanisms of neurodegenerative disorders. The first part of the book focuses on disease models and mechanisms. The areas discussed include Alzheimer's disease, Parkinson's disease, glial and neuronal death, and demyelination/remyelination. The second part concentrates on the molecular biology of neurodegeneration. The topics include molecular genetics of neurological disorders, molecular biology of recognition sites, apoptosis, and neuroimmunology and multiple sclerosis. Leading experts have been invited to give state of the art presentations including their own recent data.

P. Riederer, D. B. Calne, R. Horowski, Y. Mizuno,
W. Poewe, M. B. H. Youdim (eds.)

Advances in Research on Neurodegeneration
Volume 5

1997. 45 figures. VIII, 215 pages.
Cloth DM 198,–, öS 1386,–
ISBN 3-211-82933-4
Special edition of "Journal of Neural Transmission, Suppl. 50, 1997"

This volume focuses on brain imaging, endogenous and exogenous neurotoxins, programmed cell death, apoptosis and necrosis, and immuno-inflammatory mechanisms, infective diseases causing neurological disorders. These topics have been reviewed by invited experts and the articles give an up-to-date reflection of the state of the art in these research fields.

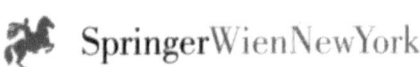

SpringerWienNewYork

Sachsenplatz 4-6, P.O.Box 89, A-1201 Wien, Fax +43-1-330 24 26
e-mail: order@springer.at, Internet: http://www.springer.at
New York, NY 10010, 175 Fifth Avenue • D-14197 Berlin, Heidelberger Platz 3
Tokyo 113, 3-13, Hongo 3-chome, Bunkyo-ku

SpringerNeurology

P. Riederer, M. B. H. Youdim (eds.)

Iron in Central Nervous System Disorders

1993. 50 figures. VII, 205 pages.
Soft cover DM 98,–, öS 686,–
ISBN 3-211-82520-7
Key Topics in Brain Research

Contents:
- Cellular and regional maintenance of iron homeostasis in the brain: normal and diseased states
- Iron deposits in brain disorders
- Brain iron and schizophrenia
- Some reflections on iron dependent free radical damage in the central nervous system
- Iron regulation of dopaminergic transmission: relevance to movement disorders
- Dopaminergic cell death in Parkinson's disease: a role of iron?
- Iron and neurotoxin intoxication: comparative in vitro and in vivo studies
- Intranigral iron infusion in rats: A progressive model for excess nigral iron levels in Parkinson's disease?
- Iron storage and transport markers in Parkinson's disease and MPTP-treated mice
- Pathogenesis of Parkinson's disease: iron and mitochondrial DNA deletion
- Consequences of intrastriatally administrated $FeCl_3$ and 6-OHDA without and after transient cerebral oligemia on behaviour and navigation
- Cytokine induced synthesis of nitric oxide from L-arginine: a cytotoxic mechanism that targets intracellular iron
- Lazaroids: potent inhibitors of iron-dependent lipid peroxidation for neurodegenerative disorders
- The treatment of iron overload – psychiatric implications
- Iron therapy: Pros and Cons

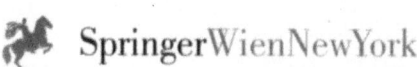

SpringerWienNewYork

Sachsenplatz 4-6, P.O.Box 89, A-1201 Wien, Fax +43-1-330 24 26
e-mail: order@springer.at, Internet: http://www.springer.at
New York, NY 10010, 175 Fifth Avenue • D-14197 Berlin, Heidelberger Platz 3
Tokyo 113, 3-13, Hongo 3-chome, Bunkyo-ku

Springer Neurology

K. A. Jellinger, G. Ladurner, M. Windisch (eds.)

New Trends in the Diagnosis and Therapy of Alzheimer's Disease

1994. 33 figures. VII, 146 pages.
Soft cover DM 130,–, öS 909,–
ISBN 3-211-82620-3
Key Topics in Brain Research

This volume based on the 2nd International Symposium of EBEWE Research Initiative in October 1993, is conceived as a review of morphological basis, diagnostic clinical and imaging techniques, cognitive assessment approaches, trial designs, outcome variables, and current trends of therapy of Alzheimer's disease. It will be of interest for all researchers, clinicians, and investigators involved in the problems of degenerative dementia disorders.

Contents:
* Synaptic pathology in the pathogenesis of Alzheimer dementia
* Classification of dementias based on functional morphology
* Computed tomography and magnetic resonance imaging in the diagnosis of Alzheimer's disease
* Diagnostic imaging techniques with special reference to PET
* Neurochemical investigations in patients with dementia of Alzheimer type and their clinical value
* Different methodological approaches for the construction of a therapy sensitive ADL scale for the assessment of Alzheimer patients
* Trial designs and outcome variables in anti-dementia drug testing
* Cognitive deterioration in old age and in the course of dementia
* NGF and Alzheimer's disease: a model for trophic factor therapy in neurodegeneration
* Efficacy of Cerebrolysin® in Alzheimer's disease

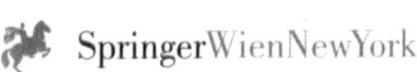

Springer Wien New York

Sachsenplatz 4-6, P.O.Box 89, A-1201 Wien, Fax +43-1-330 24 26
e-mail: order@springer.at, Internet: http://www.springer.at
New York, NY 10010, 175 Fifth Avenue • D-14197 Berlin, Heidelberger Platz 3
Tokyo 113, 3-13, Hongo 3-chome, Bunkyo-ku